Colour Aids

Sexually Transmitted Diseases

A. McMillan MD FRCP (Edin)

Consultant Physician, Department of Genito-Urinary
Medicine, Royal Infirmary, Edinburgh, UK

G. R. Scott MB ChB MRCP

Consultant Physician, Department of Genito-Urinary
Medicine, Royal Infirmary Edinburgh, UK

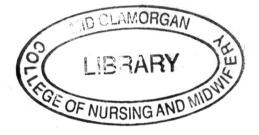

Churchill Livingstone 🏛

EDINBURGH LONDON MELBOURNE NEW YORK AND TOKYO 1991

CHURCHILL LIVINGSTONE
Medical Division of Longman Group UK Limited

Distributed in the United States of America by
Churchill Livingstone Inc., 1560 Broadway, New
York, N.Y. 10036, and by associated companies,
branches and representatives throughout the
world.

First published 1991

ISBN 0-443-04052-4

British Library Cataloguing in Publication Data

McMillan, A.
   Sexually transmitted diseases.
   1. Man. Sexually transmitted diseases
   I. Title   II. Scott, G.   III. Series
   616.951

Library of Congress Cataloging in Publication Data

McMillan, Alexander.
      Sexually transmitted diseases/A. McMillan, G. Scott.
         p.   cm.—(Colour aids)
      1. Sexually transmitted diseases—Atlases.   I. Scott, G.
   II. Title.   III. Series.
   RC200.M395   1991
   616.95'1—dc20   90-2460
                                              CIP

Produced by Longman Group (FE) Ltd
Printed in Hong Kong

Acknowledgements

We gratefully acknowledge the generosity of the following individuals in providing slides from their own collections:
Professor J. A. A. Hunter and colleagues, Department of Dermatology, University of Edinburgh; Professor C. I. Phillips, Department of Ophthalmology; Professor V. N. Sehgal, Delhi; Drs. H. Young, J. F. Peutherer, I. W. Smith, Department of Clinical Microbiology, University of Edinburgh; Dr. J. D. Oriel, Consultant Physician, University College Hospital, London; Dr. E. M. C. Dunlop, formerly Consultant Physician, Whitechapel Clinic, London; Dr. A. Blackwell, Consultant Physician, Mountpleasant Hospital, Swansea; Dr. O. P. Arya, Consultant Physician, Royal Hospital, Liverpool; Dr. J. P. Ackers, Department of Medical Protozoology, London School of Hygiene and Tropical Medicine; Dr. D. Wray, Department of Oral Medicine, Edinburgh University; Dr. C. Ludlam, Consultant Physician, Royal Infirmary of Edinburgh; Dr. D. H. H. Robertson, formerly Consultant Physician, Department of Genito-Urinary Medicine, Royal Infirmary of Edinburgh; Dr. J.G. McKenna, Senior Registrar, Department of Genito-Urinary Medicine, Royal Infirmary of Edinburgh.

We gratefully acknowledge the help of the Department of Medical Photography, Royal Infirmary of Edinburgh and our secretaries, Mrs E. J. Whittaker and Mrs L. Khosrowpour.

Contents

| # Urethritis in Men

Presenting complaint

Urethral discharge and/or dysuria.
    Additional features such as nocturia, urgency and fever should suggest the possibility of cystitis or prostatitis. A careful sexual history should be obtained.

Examination

Check for signs of other sexually transmissible conditions, e.g. rash, lymphadenopathy, pthiriasis. Examine the scrotal contents for signs of epididymo-orchitis. Examine the penis for warts or ulceration. Clean the urethral meatus before collection of material for diagnostic purposes.

Collection of specimens

A plastic loop is used when collecting exudate for microscopy and gonococcal culture. Material for culture is plated directly on to a selective medium, e.g. MNYC (Modified New York City). When direct plating is impracticable, specimens should be placed in a suitable transport medium, such as Amies or Stuart's. A cotton-wool tipped ENT swab is preferred for specimens for chlamydial diagnosis and should be passed 2–4 cm in the urethra, rotated and then withdrawn.

Diagnosis

A heat-fixed smear of exudate should be Gram-stained and examined by light microscopy. If Gram-negative diplococci (GNDC) are seen, a presumptive diagnosis of gonococcal urethritis (GU) is made although this should always be confirmed by culture.
    As microscopy will be negative in 10% of cases of GU, material for culture should be sent in every case. Non-gonococcal urethritis (NGU) is diagnosed if there are no GNDC, but ≥10 pus cells per high power field (×1000). If fewer pus cells are seen, the patient should be asked to return for an early morning smear, having held his urine overnight. Routine culture for chlamydiae is to be encouraged as this will occasionally be positive in the absence of significant numbers of pus cells. A two-glass urine test is routinely performed to differentiate anterior urethritis from posterior urethral inflammation. If both glasses remain hazy after the addition of acetic acid (to dissolve any phosphate crystals in the urine), an MSSU should also be sent for culture.

SEXUALLY TRANSMITTED DISEASES

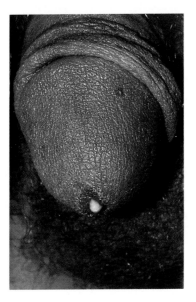

Fig. 1 Urethral discharge.

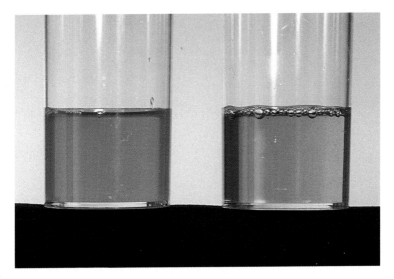

Fig. 2 Two-glass urine test—acute anterior urethritis.

2 | Vaginal Discharge

The normal vaginal discharge is composed of secretions from the upper genital tract, cervical glands, the vagina, Bartholin's glands, and the periurethral, sebaceous and apocrine glands of the vulva.

Causes

Physiological causes
Secretions increase during ovulation, immediately before menstruation, during sexual arousal and during pregnancy. A white vaginal discharge may be noted during the first 10 days of life, for about a year before the onset of the menarche; in adult women anxiety, frequent erotic stimulation, the use of the oral contraceptive and cervical ectropion may be causes.

Infections
These include:
1. *Neisseria gonorrhoeae.*
2. *Chlamydia trachomatis.*
3. *Trichomonas vaginalis.*
4. *Candida spp.*
5. Bacterial vaginosis.
6. Human papilloma virus.
7. Herpes simplex virus (HSV).

Other causes
1. Retained foreign bodies such as tampons.
2. Chemical vaginitis such as from antiseptic use.
3. Secondary infection of vaginal and cervical tears.
4. Neoplasm that may be benign (cervical polyps) or malignant.

Diagnosis

A correct diagnosis depends on the taking of a careful history, a proper examination of the lower genital tract, and the appropriate microbiological investigations. In all cases the urine should be tested for glycosuria.

SEXUALLY TRANSMITTED DISEASES

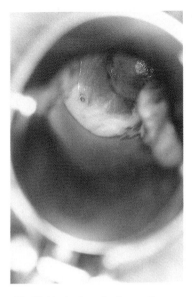

Fig. 3 Normal vaginal secretion.

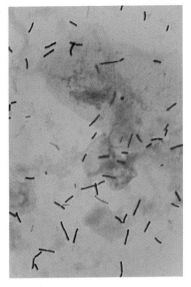

Fig. 4 Gram-stained smear of normal vaginal flora.

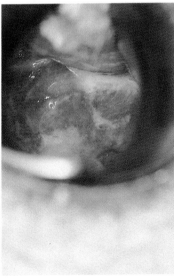

Fig. 5 Vaginitis.

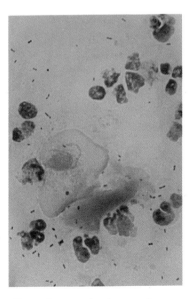

Fig. 6 Gram-stained smear from Fig. 5.

3 | Genital Ulceration

Causes and diagnosis

Bacterial infections
1. Syphilis diagnosed by dark field microscopy and serology.
2. Chancroid diagnosed by Gram-smear microscopy and by culture of *Haemophilus ducreyi*.
3. *Lymphogranuloma venereum* diagnosed by culture of *C. trachomatis* or serology.
4. *Granuloma inguinale* diagnosed by Giemsa-smear microscopy or biopsy.
5. Pyogenic infection diagnosed by bacterial culture.
6. Tuberculosis (rare) diagnosed by biopsy or culture.

Viral Infections
1. Herpes simplex virus diagnosed by culture (send specimen in Hank's viral transport medium) or serology.
2. Herpes zoster: dermatomal distribution; diagnosis by culture.

Protozoal infestation
Entaemoeba histolytica (rare): histological diagnosis.

Multisystem conditions
1. Erythema multiforme.
2. Behçet's syndrome.
3. Fixed drug eruptions.

Other causes
1. Chemical irritation with a history of contact.
2. Trauma: diagnosis made on history.
3. Malignancy: histological diagnosis.

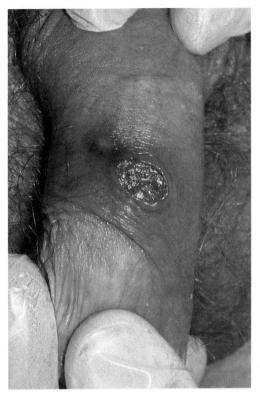

Fig. 7 Genital ulcer—pyogenic.

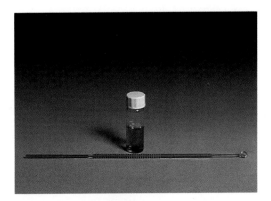

Fig. 8 Hank's viral transport medium.

4 | Gonorrhoea (1)

Aetiology

Gonorrhoea is caused by the bacterium *Neisseria gonorrhoeae* (commonly referred to as the gonococcus) that infects mucosal surfaces of the genitourinary tract, rectum and pharynx.

Epidemiology

Gonorrhoea is transmitted almost exclusively by sexual contact. In the UK and USA it is one of the most prevalent infections after the childhood exanthemata. Incidence rates fell after the Second World War with the advent of antibiotics, then rose through the 1960s. The incidence has been falling since the mid-1970s. Rectal gonorrhoea in the male (reflecting homosexual contact) has fallen substantially in recent years as a result of changing sexual behaviour in the face of the epidemic of HIV infection. β-lactamase-producing strains of the organism are prevalent in South East Asia and in West Africa.

Clinical features

In males
Urethral infection is symptomatic in 90% of cases. A purulent or mucopurulent discharge and/or dysuria develops after a prepatent period of 3–5 days (range 2–14 days). Complications are relatively rare, as patients tend to seek medical advice before these develop. Infection may spread to involve parafrenal (Tyson's) glands, the epididymis, prostate, glans penis and median raphe. Late complications such as urethral stricture are now extremely rare.

Unilateral epididymo-orchitis is the most common complication, and prompt diagnosis and treatment is essential to prevent abscess formation. Disseminated gonococcal infection (DGI) is rare.

Pharyngeal infection as a result of orogenital contact rarely produces symptoms.

Rectal infection is also usually symptomless although a few patients may complain of anal discharge, pain and tenesmus. Proctoscopy may reveal no clinical features of proctitis.

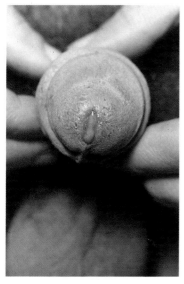

Fig. 9 Gonococcal urethritis.

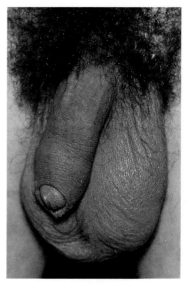

Fig. 10 Gonococcal epididymo-orchitis.

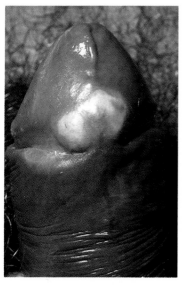

Fig. 11 Gonococcal infection of the parafrenal (Tyson's) glands.

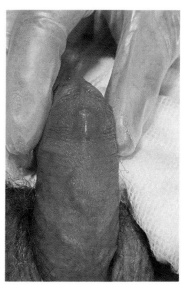

Fig. 12 Gonococcal infection of the median raphe.

4 | Gonorrhoea (2)

Clinical features

In adult females
Genital infection in the female is symptomless in over 70% of cases. The cervix is involved in 85–90% of cases, but the resultant discharge is profuse enough to be recognised in only 10%. Urethral infection (65–70%) is usually symptomless although there may be occasional dysuria and urinary frequency. Anorectal infection (30–50%) is almost invariably symptomless. The vagina is not infected. Pharyngeal infection as a result of fellatio is usually asymptomatic.

Complications: involvement of the greater vestibular (Bartholin's) gland may result in abscess formation. Ascending infection from the cervix resulting in gonococcal salpingitis occurs in 10% cases. The presentation is usually acute with lower abdominal pain and fever. Clinical signs include pyrexia, lower abdominal tenderness, guarding, adnexal swelling and pain on cervical excitation during bimanual examination, raised white cell count and ESR. Irreversible tubal damage may occur within 72 hours and long-term sequelae include ectopic (tubal) pregnancy, and infertility if infection is bilateral. Inflammation of the liver capsule (perihepatitis) following spillage of infected tubal secretion into the peritoneum is a rare complication.

Disseminated gonococcal infection: haematogenous dissemination occurs in less than 1% of cases. Most patients with DGI have no genitourinary symptoms; the syndrome is more common in women. The main features are pyrexia, a vasculitic rash and arthropathy, which is usually confined to a single large joint such as a knee or elbow. Gonococcal culture from joint aspirate and blood is frequently negative, and the diagnosis is made from material obtained from the genital tract.

SEXUALLY TRANSMITTED DISEASES

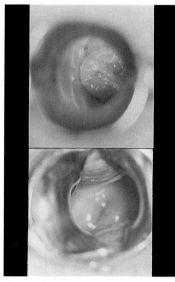

Fig. 13 Gonococcal cervicitis.

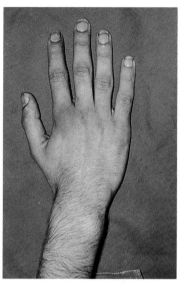

Fig. 14 Gonococcal arthritis.

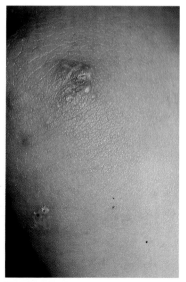

Fig. 15 Papulopustule of disseminated gonococcal infection.

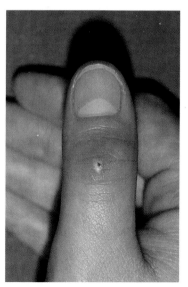

Fig. 16 Papulopustule of disseminated gonococcal infection.

4 | Gonorrhoea (3)

Clinical features

In children
Ophthalmia neonatorum: gonococcal cervicitis in pregnancy may lead to infection of the neonatal conjunctivae during birth. A purulent discharge usually develops within 48 hours. If treatment is delayed, corneal scarring may result.

Vulvovaginitis: the soft stratified squamous epithelium of prepubertal girls is susceptible to gonococcal infection. Vaginal discharge and vulval erythema are therefore more common than in adult women. Historically, the mode of acquisition has been considered to be accidental contamination, but this view has fallen into disfavour with the suspicion that up to 95% of cases may represent sexual abuse.

Diagnosis

In men, a Gram-stained smear of urethral exudate should be examined microscopically for GNDCs, although every case should be confirmed by culture. As microscopy may be negative, material for culture should always be sent in a suitable transport medium such as Amies or Stuart's. Gonococci are cultured on a selective medium such as MNYC in a CO_2 enriched atmosphere, with identification of suspected colonies by oxidase reaction, sugar utilisation tests, coagglutination and immunofluorescence.

SEXUALLY TRANSMITTED DISEASES

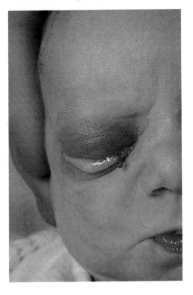

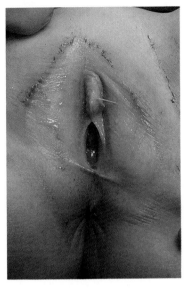

Fig. 17 Gonococcal ophthalmia neonatorum.

Fig. 18 Gonococcal vulvovaginitis.

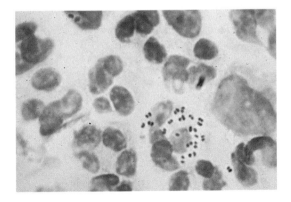

Fig. 19 Gram-negative diplococci in urethral smear.

4 | Gonorrhoea (4)

Diagnosis

When oral or anal intercourse is suspected, material for culture should be taken from the pharynx and rectum on two occasions as infection of these sites is more difficult to diagnose. In females, microscopy of cervical material will be positive in less than 50% of cases. As the urethra and rectum are frequently colonised by the gonococcus (and may be the only affected sites) material for culture should be obtained from these sites in addition to the cervix. Culture should be repeated at least once before gonococcal infection is excluded. A high vaginal swab will fail to diagnose 50% of infections.

Treatment

Single-dose therapy is adequate for uncomplicated genital infection in either sex. Clinical practice varies but generally ampicillin or amoxycillin with probenecid is prescribed. More prolonged courses of 5–7 days are required for rectal infection in either sex. Where infection is complicated parenteral penicillin for several days is indicated. Other antimicrobial agents such as cefuroxime, spectinomycin and ciprofloxacin may be indicated in areas where gonococcal strains resistant to penicillin are prevalent or in individual cases of pencillin hypersensitivity.

Co-infection with chlamydiae is present in 40% of heterosexual patients, and it is thus common practice to prescribe a course of tetracycline or erythromycin to be taken after completion of therapy for gonococcal infection. Contact tracing is essential.

At least two tests of cure should be performed in the female. In the male with gonococcal urethritis the disappearance of symptoms may be regarded as evidence of cure.

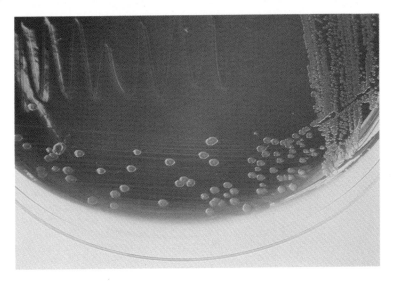

Fig. 20 Colonies of *N. gonorrhoeae* on MNYC medium.

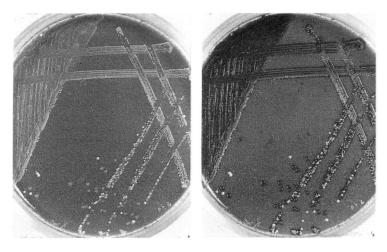

Fig. 21 Positive oxidase reaction with Neisseriae (White colonies are *S. epidermidis*.)

5 Non-specific Genital Infection (NSGI) (1)

Aetiology

Chlamydia trachomatis causes 50−70% of cases of NSGI, which in males is referred to as non-gonococcal urethritis (NGU). *C. trachomatis* may be divided immunologically into a number of serotypes (serovars). Types A, B and C are associated with the ocular infection trachoma, types L 1−3 are associated with lymphogranuloma venereum, whereas the oculogenital serovars D−K are associated with NGU. The role of other organisms is less certain, but *Ureaplasma urealyticum*, *Mycoplasma genitalium*, and *Bacteroides* species may account for 10−20%. Occasional cases are due to infection with HSV, *Trichomonas vaginalis* and coliforms. In a significant proportion no organism is identified. Such cases may represent infection with unknown agents or be non-infectious, i.e. true 'non-specific urethritis'.

Epidemiology

NSGI is three times as common as gonococcal infection in the UK, with similar prevalence rates worldwide. Precise epidemiological observation has been hampered by difficulties in diagnosing chlamydial infection.

Clinical features

In males
Chlamydial infection of the urethra is symptomless in approximately 25% of cases. In the remaining 75% and in cases of non-chlamydial NGU, the prepatent period is 1−4 weeks, following which a mucoid or mucopurulent discharge and/or dysuria develops. Symptoms are usually less marked than with gonococcal urethritis, but there is considerable overlap and differentiation on clinical grounds alone is not advised. Chlamydial infection of the rectum is usually symptomless, although infection with L 1−3 serovars may result in acute proctitis.

Complications: the main one is epididymo-orchitis, of which chlamydiae are the commonest cause in young sexually active men. A role for chlamydiae in prostatitis has been postulated but not substantiated. Auto-inoculation may result in conjunctivitis. Reiter's syndrome is discussed on pp. 21−26.

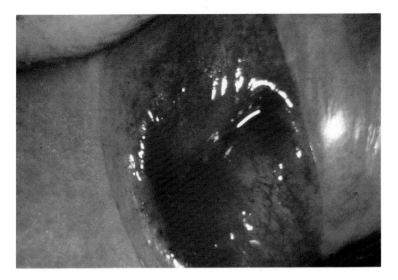

Fig. 22 Non-gonococcal urethritis.

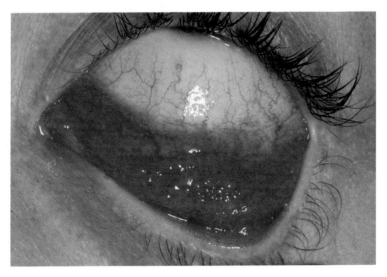

Fig. 23 Chlamydial conjunctivitis.

5 | Non-specific Genital Infection (2)

In females
Chlamydial infection of the cervix is usually symptomless, although examination may reveal a follicular or 'cobblestone' appearance. About one-third of patients complain of increased vaginal discharge. Urethral infection (present in 10−20%) may result in dysuria and/or urinary frequency. Ascending infection may result in salpingitis for which chlamydiae are the single most common cause, accounting for approximately 30% of cases admitted to gynaecology units. The abdominal pain and degree of systemic upset are usually less marked than with gonococcal salpingitis. Spillage of infected material from the salpinges with transcoelomic spread to the liver capsule may cause perihepatitis (Fitz-Hugh-Curtis syndrome). This results in right hypochondrial pain and tenderness which may be mistaken for cholecystitis. A high index of suspicion is required as the accompanying salpingitis may be covert. Infertility due to bilateral tubal obstruction is a frequent complication of untreated and recurrent chlamydial salpingitis.

In children
Chlamydial infection of the birth canal leads to neonatal conjunctivitis in 50% of those exposed. Symptoms that develop about 1 week after birth are usually mild and self-limiting. Aspiration of infected material results in pneumonia in about 10% of neonates exposed. This usually occurs at 2−3 months of age, and whilst not life threatening, may result in significant lung damage. It is also postulated that the neonatal vagina may become infected at birth and that this infection may not be detected for several years. The possibility of sexual abuse in such cases however, should always be carefully considered.

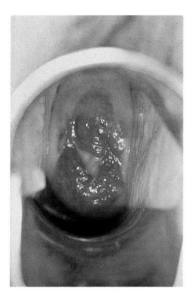

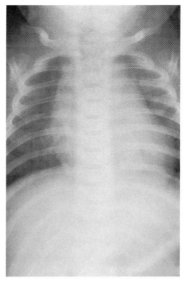

Fig. 24 Chlamydial cervicitis.

Fig. 25 Chlamydial pneumonitis in an infant.

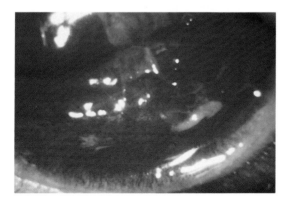

Fig. 26 Chlamydial conjunctivitis in a neonate.

5 | Non-specific Genital Infection (3)

Diagnosis

Non-gonococcal urethritis in men implies that the diagnosis is one of exclusion, and essentially this is the case. NGU is diagnosed if a Gram's-stained smear from the urethra reveals numerous pus cells but no Gram-negative diplococci, and gonococcal culture is negative. The precise number of pus cells regarded as significant varies among centres, but the authors regard $\geqslant 10$ pus cells per high-power field as indicative of urethritis. If facilities allow, the diagnosis may be backed up by detection of chlamydiae.

No such clear-cut guidelines for the diagnosis of NSGI exist in women. The decision to treat is often based on epidemiological grounds backed up by screening for chlamydial infection.

Chlamydial infection
Chlamydiae are intracellular bacteria, so care is required to ensure that adequate material is obtained from the urethra or cervix for diagnostic purposes.

Chlamydial isolation may be attempted in tissue-cell cultures for which clinical specimens should be placed in a special transport medium such as 2SP. Alternatively, chlamydial antigens may be detected by immunofluorescence or Elisa.

Treatment

Oxytetracycline is usually effective. Minocycline and doxycycline are acceptable (albeit more expensive) alternatives. Tetracyclines are contraindicated in pregnancy; erythromycin is an alternative for the treatment of women. Contact tracing is essential. Epidemiological treatment of female partners of men with NGU is widely favoured.

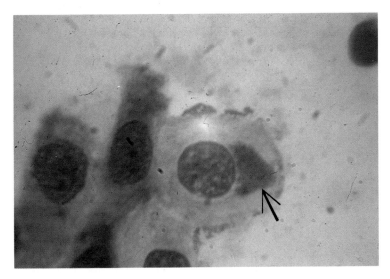

Fig. 27 Inclusion bodies of chlamydiae (Giemsa stain).

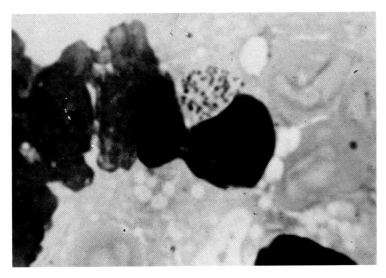

Fig. 28 Reticulate bodies of chlamydiae.

6 | Reiter's Syndrome (1)

Definition

In 1916 the triad of urethritis, arthritis and conjunctivitis was described by Hans Reiter. The major component of the syndrome is the arthropathy, and the other features are not invariably present. The syndrome may follow either gastrointestinal infection (due to salmonella, shigella, yersinia or campylobacter) or genitourinary infection (due to chlamydiae and possibly other agents). The acronyms EARA (enterically acquired reactive arthritis) and SARA (sexually acquired reactive arthritis) have also been proposed for these two forms.

Genetic factors

The histocompatibility antigen HLA B27 is present in up to 80% of patients with Reiter's syndrome. The syndrome overlaps with ankylosing spondylitis that is also associated with HLA B27. The male : female ratio is approximately 50 : 1.

Clinical features

The post-venereal form is more commonly seen in the UK, and follows NGU in approximately 1% of cases. The onset is acute, occurring 2–3 weeks post infection. A few joints only are affected, classically knees and ankles, although other large joints may be involved. Joint rupture may occur occasionally.

Sacro-iliitis is common whereas inflammation of the small joints of hands and feet is not. Urethritis is indistinguishable from other forms of NGU. Conjunctivitis is present in one-third of cases and is bilateral.

Other common features include tenosynovitis (especially of the Achilles' tendon), plantar fasciitis, circinate balanitis and keratoderma blennorrhagica. Less common are uveitis, lesions of the oral mucosa, carditis, glomerulonephritis and thrombophlebitis.

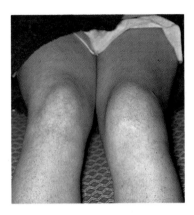

Fig. 29 Arthritis of knee joint.

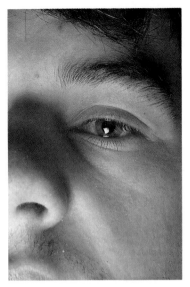

Fig. 30 Mild Conjunctivitis.

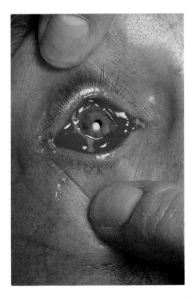

Fig. 31 Severe conjunctivitis.

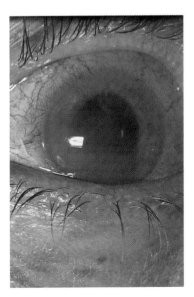

Fig. 32 Anterior uveitis.

Differential diagnosis

Gonococcal arthritis must be excluded by collection of appropriate specimens for gonococcal culture. It should be noted however, that as gonococcal and chlamydial infections frequently co-exist, 5% of patients with RS initially present with gonorrhoea. Rheumatoid arthritis is usually excluded by the pattern of joint involvement, the presence of urethritis, and the absence of IgM rheumatoid factor. Ankylosing spondylitis and other seronegative arthropathies may be more difficult to exclude, but the presence of urethritis and acute onset of symptoms should be diagnostic.

Diagnosis

There is no diagnostic test for Reiter's syndrome and the diagnosis is made on clinical grounds alone. The ESR is usually raised and HLA B27 is often present.

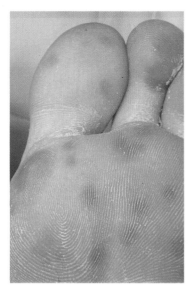

Fig. 33 Keratoderma
blennorrhagica.

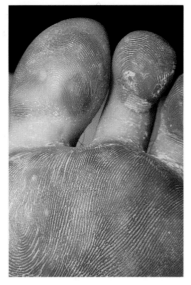

Fig. 34 Keratoderma
blennorrhagica.

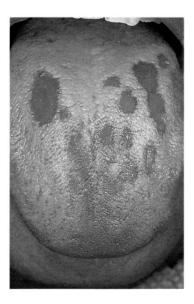

Fig. 35 Mucosal lesions of the
tongue.

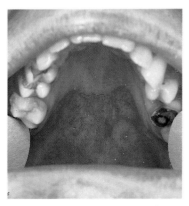

Fig. 36 Petechial lesions of the
palate.

Treatment

The urethritis is managed conventionally with tetracycline and usually clears promptly. As the arthropathy usually resolves within 3−6 months, symptomatic therapy alone is indicated. Aspirin may be sufficient to control joint inflammation, but commonly a more powerful anti-inflammatory drug such as naproxen or indomethacin is required. Acutely inflamed joints should be rested, and physiotherapy instituted to prevent muscle wasting. Where a large effusion has accumulated in a joint, aspiration of fluid followed by instillation of methylprednisolone or indomethacin will give considerable relief.

Conjunctivitis may be treated with saline lavage or beta-methasone eye drops. Uveitis should be managed in conjunction with an ophthalmologist.

Circinate balanitis is treated with hydrocortisone cream.

Keratoderma is difficult to treat but is self-limiting.

Prognosis

The majority of cases resolve within 3−6 months. Recurrences, however, are common. In some patients the arthropathy evolves to a chronic condition indistinguishable from ankylosing spondylitis.

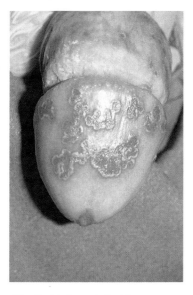

Fig. 37 Circinate balanitis.

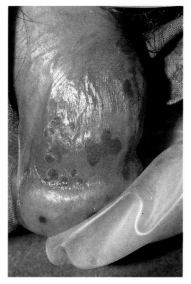

Fig. 38 Circinate balanitis.

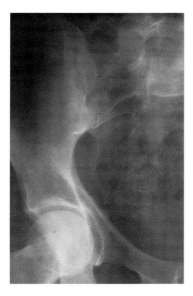

Fig. 39 Sacro-iliitis.

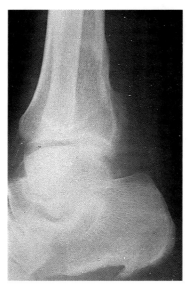

Fig. 40 Plantar spur.

Syphilis (1)

Aetiology

Syphilis is caused by the bacterium *Treponema pallidum ssp pallidum* which is spread principally by sexual contact but which can be acquired congenitally.

Epidemiology

In the UK the incidence of early syphilis fell sharply in the immediate post-war years and has remained constant since then. Over the past 20 years more than 50% of male cases had been acquired homosexually. The incidence of late-stage and congenital infection remains low. Syphilis is still prevalent in the developing world.

Although individuals with syphilis of more than 4 years' duration cease to be infective sexually, a pregnant woman can transmit the infection to her child during the later stages of pregnancy.

Acquired syphilis

Clinical features

Primary syphilis
After a prepatent period of about 3 weeks (range 10–90 days), a dull red papule that soon ulcerates develops at the site of inoculation of the treponeme. The ulcer (chancre) is single, painless, and well-demarcated. It is indurated but not tender; the full, red, flat surface may be covered with a flat crust. Serous fluid but not blood exudes from the surface.

The lesion may be found anywhere on the external genitalia or on the cervix uteri. Anal chancres may be atypical and resemble fissures. Oral lesions are rare. Bilateral inguinal lymph-node enlargement occurs.

The lesion heals within 3–8 weeks leaving a thin scar.

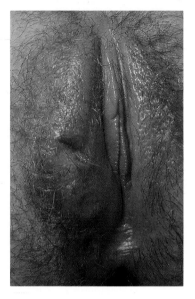

Fig. 41 Vulval chancres.

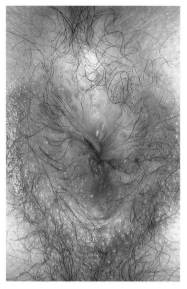

Fig. 42 Chancre of anal canal.

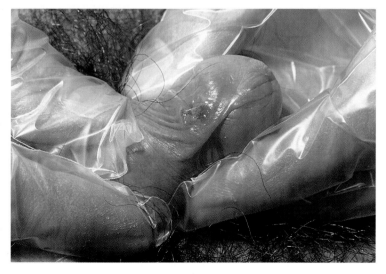

Fig. 43 Penile chancre.

Syphilis (2)

Acquired syphilis (contd)

Secondary syphilis
Signs of this stage develop 7–10 weeks after infection, and in some patients the primary lesion is still present. The clinical features may appear and regress at intervals over a 2-year period. The patient complains of malaise, mild fever, headache, a skin rash that may be mildly pruritic, hoarseness, swollen lymph nodes, patchy or diffuse hair loss, arthralgia and bone pain.

Skin lesions are noticed in over 80% of cases. The earliest lesions are rose-pink macules that are symmetrically distributed over the body. A symmetrically distributed papular rash is more commonly seen. Initially the lesions have a shiny surface but later scaling occurs. Papules may be found in the nasolabial folds, below the hairline, and on the palms and soles. In moist areas such as the perianal region, the papules are hypertrophic and may be eroded (condylomata lata). Involvement of the hair follicles may result in patchy hair loss. In the later stages of secondary syphilis the papules become fewer and are distributed asymmetrically. Condylomata lata may be the only feature at this stage. Lesions heal without scarring but depigmentation may occur.

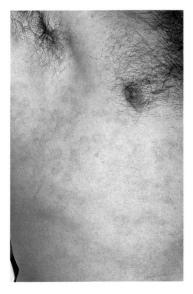

Fig. 44 Early macular rash.

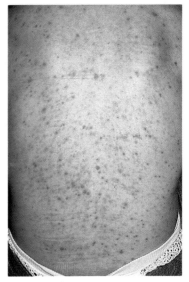

Fig. 45 Maculopapular rash.

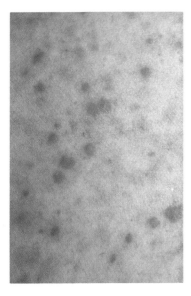

Fig. 46 Maculopapular rash (close-up).

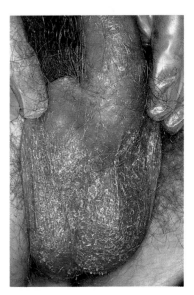

Fig. 47 Psoriasiform rash.

Acquired syphilis (contd)

Secondary syphilis (contd)
Mucosal lesions occur in 30% of patients. They
are oval superficial ulcers covered with a grey
membrane; adjacent lesions may coalesce. They
are found on the tonsils, buccal mucosa, tongue,
larynx and genitalia.

Other features of secondary syphilis include
generalised lymphadenopathy, and less
commonly, hepatitis, glomerulonephritis,
choroidoretinitis, meningoencephalitis, and
periostitis.

The differential diagnosis of secondary syphilis
includes drug eruptions, measles, rubella,
infectious mononucleosis, pityriasis rosea,
psoriasis, lichen planus, pityriasis lichenoides,
anogenital warts, herpes simplex infection,
trichophytides, aphthous ulceration and keratotic
eczema.

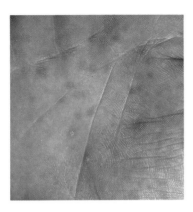

Fig. 48 Palmar lesions.

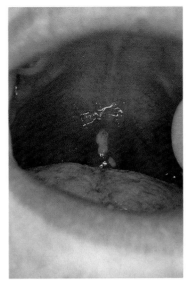

Fig. 49 Mucous patch.

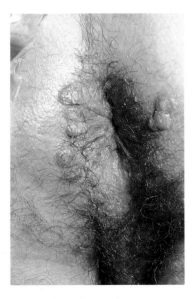

Fig. 50 Condylomata lata.

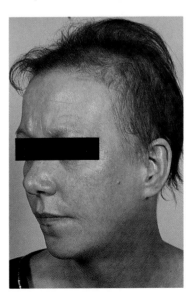

Fig. 51 Diffuse alopecia.

Acquired syphilis (contd)

Clinical features (contd)

Latent syphilis
The lesions of secondary syphilis heal and the disease becomes latent, being detectable only by serological testing. The distinction between early-latent and late-latent disease is arbitrary, but syphilis of over 2 years' duration is considered to be late.

Gummatous syphilis
When host resistance to the treponeme fails in the late stages of infection, localised gummatous lesions (syphilitic granulation tissue) develop. The lesion is a single punched ulcer of the skin, especially of the scalp, upper outer aspect of the leg or the sternoclavicular region. The mouth or pharynx may be affected. Diffuse infiltration of the tongue with chronic superficial glossitis on which leukoplakia may subsequently develop may occur. Gummatous periostitis or osteitis may be features. Generally there is a good response to treatment.

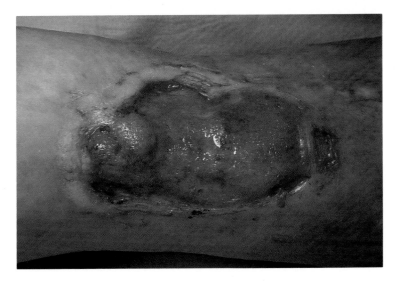

Fig. 52 Gumma of leg.

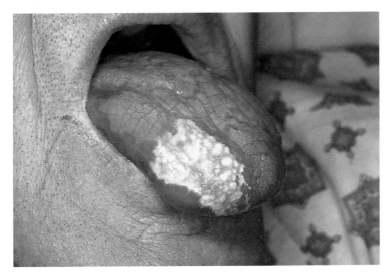

Fig. 53 Leukoplakia of tongue.

Acquired syphilis (contd)

Clinical features (contd)

Neurosyphilis
This may be symptomless and detectable only by the examination of the CSF. The clinical course may be accelerated if there is concomitant HIV infection. Meningovascular syphilis may produce headache, cranial nerve palsies, and if the cerebral vessels are affected, focal signs and mental deterioration. General paralysis of the insane (GPI) can develop 7–15 years after infection; dementia is the usual presenting feature. In tabes dorsalis, the degenerative lesions are concentrated on the dorsal columns of the lumbosacral and lower thoracic levels of the spinal cord. Lightning pains, paraesthesiae, ataxia, disturbances of bladder and bowel control, and crises (paroxysmal painful disorders of the viscera) are all features. There is muscle hypotonia with diminution of lower limb reflexes, and optic atrophy. Trophic ulcers may develop on the soles and neuropathic joints (Charcot's) may occur in the lower limbs.

The Argyll-Robertson pupil is the characteristic pupillary change in all forms of late neurosyphilis. It is small, constant in size, reacting to accommodation but not to light, patchily depigmented, and dilating slowly to mydriatics. Other abnormalities are also found.

Cardiovascular syphilis
Aortitis, especially of the aortic ring and ascending part of the aorta with resulting destruction of elastic tissue, may produce aortic incompetence or aneurysm formation.

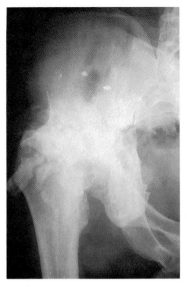

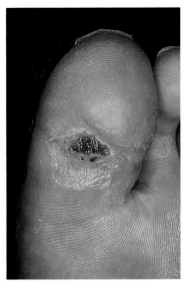

Fig. 54 Neuropathic (Charcot's) joint.

Fig. 55 Perforating ulcer.

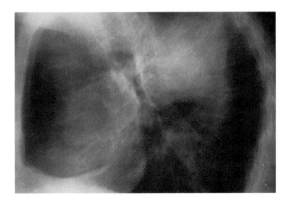

Fig. 56 Aortic aneurysm.

Congenital syphilis

**Clinical
features**

Early
Signs are in the neonate who is often premature
or of low birth weight. The skin is wrinkled and
there is a bullous rash on the soles and palms; the
liver is enlarged. Characteristic features of early
disease develop 2–12 weeks after birth when the
child fails to thrive. There is a symmetrically
distributed macular, papular or papulosquamous
rash, especially around the mouth. Deep fissures
around the orifices heal with scarring (rhagades).
Nail atrophy is common. The lesions heal within
the first year, but there may be recurrences during
the second year. Rhinitis is common and nasal
deformity may result from arrested development
of the nasal bones. Periostitis may be apparent
radiologically, dactylitis may occur, and
choroidoretinitis may be a feature. Generalised
lymphadenopathy, hepatic and splenic
enlargement are common. Anaemia and
thrombocytopenia can occur. Meningitis is
common.

Late
After their second birthday infected children are
said to have late-stage disease. There may be no
clinical features (latent), or the features listed on
p. 39 may occur.

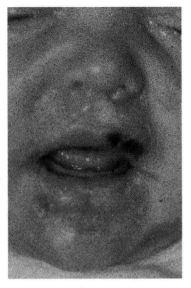 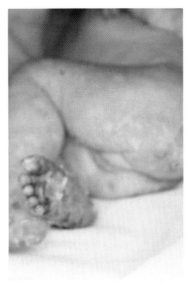

Fig. 57 Congenital syphilitic rhinitis (snuffles). Due to the rarity of this condition an old slide has been used. We apologize for the quality of reproduction.

Fig. 58 Rash of congenital syphilis.

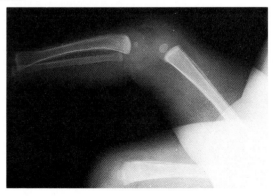

Fig. 59 Periostitis.

Congenital syphilis (contd)

Interstitial keratitis: develops between the ages of 6 and 14 years. There is pain in the affected eye and photophobia. Central corneal haziness occurs. Ultimately both eyes are affected. There is improvement over 12–18 months but scarring often results.

Hypertrophic osteoperiostitis: can be either diffuse or localised and principally affects the tibiae. Lesions develop between the ages of 5 and 20 years. Gummatous lesions of the hard and soft palates and nasal septum result in scarring and possibly perforation.

Clutton's joints: may develop between the ages of 5 and 10 years. There is acute onset of painless swelling of the knee joints. Resolution is full.

Sensory neural deafness: may be a feature, but juvenile GPI and tabes dorsalis are rare. Paroxysmal cold haemoglobinuria is also rare.

Stigmata: lesions of early and late congenital syphilis heal leaving scars (stigmata). Facial stigmata include 'saddle-nose' deformity and a high arched palate. The molars may have a constricted occlusal surface (Moon's molars) and the incisors may be small and peg-like with a notched edge (Hutchinson's incisors). Rhagades, atrophic nails, choroidal scarring, corneal opacities, including 'ghost vessels', bony deformities such as 'sabre tibia', optic atrophy, and eighth-nerve deafness may be noted.

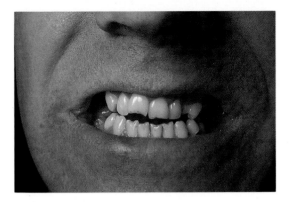

Fig. 60 Hutchinson's incisors.

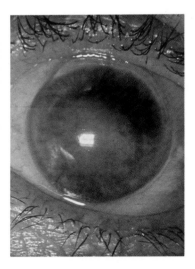

Fig. 61 Interstitial keratitis.

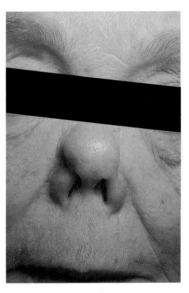

Fig. 62 Saddle-nose deformity.

7 | Syphilis (8)

Diagnosis

Treponema pallidum can be detected in the serum from the base of a chancre by dark-field microscopy or direct immunofluorescence. Serological tests form the principal diagnostic methods for all other stages of the infection. A cardiolipin antibody test (e.g. Venereal Diseases Research Laboratory test—VDRL) and a specific treponemal antibody test (e.g. *T. pallidum* haemagglutination test—TPHA) are used for screening. A positive result in either is confirmed using the fluorescent treponemal antibody-absorption test (FTA-Abs). This is also the most sensitive test for early disease. In untreated infections the TPHA and FTA-Abs remain positive for life (IgG antibodies). Over time the VDRL becomes negative in one-third of cases. Specific IgM can be detected in untreated disease. With successful treatment, the VDRL becomes negative within about one year of successful treatment of early syphilis; the TPHA and FTA-Abs may remain positive for years. Persistence of cardiolipin and treponemal antibodies is common after treatment of late-stage disease. Neurosyphilis is diagnosed by finding treponemal antibodies in the CSF. The detection of 19S (IgM) antibodies in the baby's blood is the most reliable test for congenital infection. Serum from patients with the endemic treponematoses yields positive results in the above tests.

Treatment

Penicillin is the treatment of choice. In individuals with penicillin hypersensitivity, tetracyclines or erythromycin are alternatives. The Jarisch-Herxheimer reaction may occur within 4 hours of treatment of early and neurosyphilis.

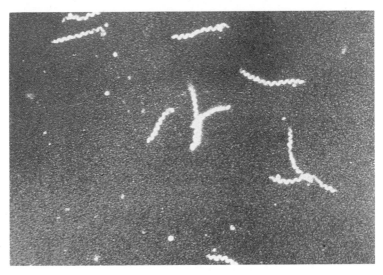

Fig. 63 *T. pallidum* by dark-ground microscopy.

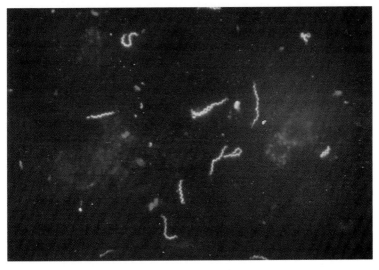

Fig. 64 *T. pallidum* by direct immunofluorescence.

8 | Genital Warts (1)

Aetiology

Caused by the DNA-containing human papilloma virus (HPV). Although the virus cannot be cultured in vitro, different types can be identified by DNA-DNA hybridisation methods. Genital warts are most commonly caused by types 6b and 11, but types 16 and 18 are sometimes found either singly or with the former types.

Epidemiology

The incidence of genital warts in the UK has been increasing over the past 15 years. Most individuals have acquired the virus through sexual contact, but although their presence may indicate sexual abuse, in children these warts may be acquired non-sexually. Laryngeal papillomata in children may result from infection as the child passes down the birth canal of an infected mother. Some infected individuals have subclinical lesions that can only be identified by colposcopy; they may represent a reservoir of infection in the community. One-third of patients with genital warts have a concurrent sexually transmitted disease. There is an association between certain HPV types (16, 18, 33) and malignant disease of the genital tract. As healthy individuals can harbour these types, cofactors are probably important in carcinogenesis.

Clinical features

The prepatent period is very variable and difficult to define; warts may develop up to 2 years from contact with an infected person.

In males
Hyperplastic condylomata acuminata are found in the coronal sulcus, on the inner aspect of the prepuce, at the urethral meatus, in the perianal region and within the anal canal. Sessile and plane warts may be found on the shaft of the penis.

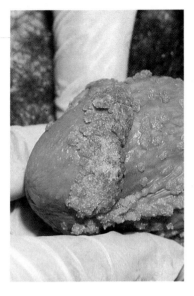

Fig. 65 Subpreputial warts.

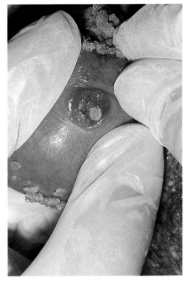

Fig. 66 Intrameatal warts.

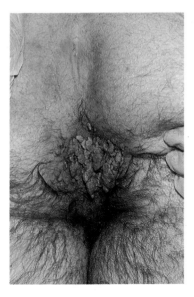

Fig. 67 Perianal warts.

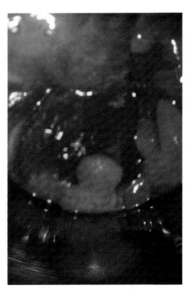

Fig. 68 Intra-anal warts.

8 | Genital Warts (2)

Clinical features (contd)

In females

In women, condylomata acuminata are found at the introitus, on the labia minora and majora, perineum, vagina, perianal region, urethra and cervix. Although the cervix may appear normal macroscopically, by colposcopy, after the application of 5% acetic acid, slightly raised aceto-white areas may be seen in some women with HPV infection of that site.

Dysplastic-like changes are found in cervical biopsies from up to 50% of women with genital warts. Although spontaneous regression of the milder degrees of dysplasia has been reported, the natural history of such changes is unknown. Rarely, in both sexes, intra-oral condylomata occur.

Diagnosis

The diagnosis is clinical. Conditions that require differentiation include penile papillae, molluscum contagiosum, condylomata lata, and early squamous cell carcinoma.

Treatment

In the absence of specific antiviral therapy, treatment is aimed at controlling growth of the warts and reducing the risk of sepsis. Podophyllin resin suspended in liquid paraffin or ethanol, or, perhaps better, podophyllotoxin, is applied topically at regular intervals until the lesions regress. Its use on the cervix, vagina or within the anal canal should be avoided, and as the drug can be absorbed systemically it should not be used in pregnancy. Cryotherapy, electrocautery or diathermy, and scissor excision are used also in treatment.

Annual cervical cytology is recommended in women who have or have had genital warts. Sexual contacts should be examined.

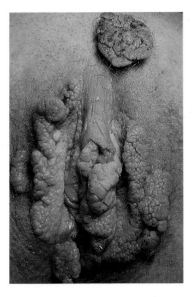

Fig. 69 Vulval warts.

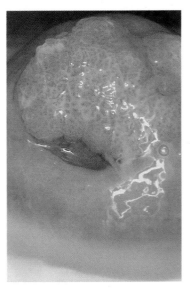

Fig. 70 Cervical condyloma.

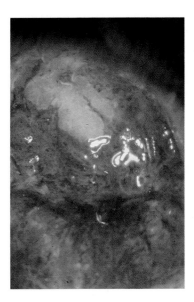

Fig. 71 Aceto-white areas of the cervix with HPV infection.

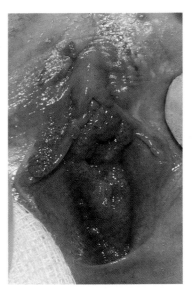

Fig. 72 Prepubertal introital warts.

9 | Genital Herpes (1)

Aetiology

There are two types of the DNA-containing herpes simplex virus—types 1 and 2.

Pathogenesis

At the site of entry into the body through the skin or mucosae there is multiplication of virus with infection of nerve endings. Nucleocapsid is transported via the axon to the dorsal root ganglia where further multiplication occurs. Infectious virions then migrate centrifugally to the surface. After resolution of the primary infection, latency is established. Reactivation may occur with or without clinical disease.

Epidemiology

Over the past 15 years the prevalence of genital herpes in developed countries has increased. Although lesions at this site are associated classically with HSV 2, 15–30% of isolates are HSV 1. Symptomless excretion probably is important in maintaining the infection in the community. A previous HSV 1 infection may protect against acquisition of a clinically apparent HSV 2 infection.

Clinical features

Primary infections: genital lesions are accompanied by systemic symptoms—fever, headache, malaise and myalgia. Painful or itchy lesions develop with dysuria and sometimes a urethral or vaginal discharge. Multiple papules, vesicles or pustules that ulcerate appear on the genitalia. After a variable period, crusting and healing occurs but new lesions may form. There is inguinal lymphadenitis. Lesions usually heal within 3–4 weeks. Extragenital lesions, and sacral cadiculitis may occur. Proctitis may result from anal intercourse. HSV 1 primary infections tend to be less severe than those associated with HSV 2.

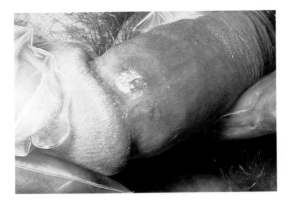

Fig. 73 Herpetic ulcer on the penis.

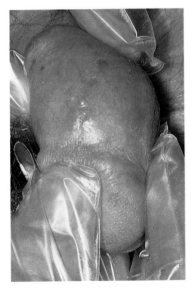

Fig. 74 Herpetic vesicle on the penis.

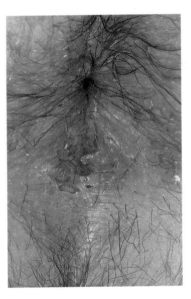

Fig. 75 Perianal herpes in a homosexual man.

9 | Genital Herpes (2)

Clinical features (contd)

Initial infections: in patients with initial infections (i.e. persons who have clinical or serological evidence of prior HSV infection) the disease is milder than in those suffering primary infections.

Recurrent infections: the lesions of recurrent herpes resemble those of the initial episode but are localised to the genitalia, are of lesser extent, heal more quickly and are not associated with systemic features. There may be prodromal symptoms e.g. tingling in the area. There is individual variation in the frequency of recurrences, but they are more likely in persons with HSV 2 infections. Symptomless recurrences are well-documented.

Diagnosis

Diagnosis is by viral isolation in tissue culture, or antigen detection in material from lesions. Serology may be useful in primary infections.

Treatment

Acyclovir given orally is the treatment of choice for primary and initial herpes; it may be used also in recurrences but the effects are not so obvious. In individuals with particularly frequent recurrences or in immunocompromised patients, prophylactic use of the drug may be necessary. Drug resistance is very rare.

Genital herpes in pregnancy
Primary HSV 2 infection during pregnancy, particularly during the third trimester, may be associated with prematurity and growth retardation. Infection during parturition is associated with high neonatal mortality. This can be prevented by delivery by Caesarean section before membrane rupture.
   The risk of neonatal herpes is much lower in women with recurrent disease.

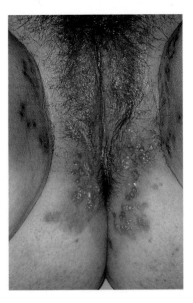

Fig. 76 Herpetic ulceration of the vulva.

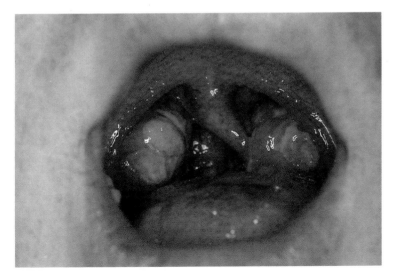

Fig. 77 Herpetic ulceration of the tonsils.

10 | Molluscum contagiosum

Aetiology

Caused by a virus of the DNA-containing poxvirus group.

Epidemiology

Over the past decade the incidence in the UK has been increasing. The virus is transmitted by personal contact, including sexual, or by fomites.

Clinical features

After a prepatent period of 15–50 days, pearly, raised, firm, hemispherical papules about 2–5 mm in diameter and with an umbilicated centre appear either singly or in groups on the affected area. Although they may persist for many months, spontaneous regression usually occurs.

Diagnosis

This is clinical, but can be confirmed by electron microscopy of material from the core.

Treatment

Piercing with a sharpened orange stick that has been dipped in tincture of iodine, cryotherapy, or electrocautery are effective. Sexual partners should be examined also.

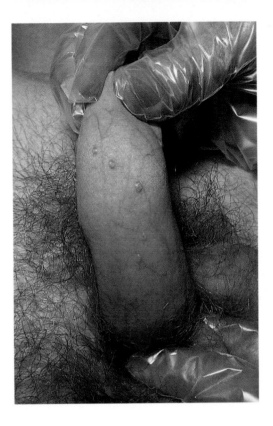

Fig. 78 Molluscum contagiosum of the shaft of the
penis.

11 | Hepatitis B

Aetiology

Caused by the DNA-containing hepatitis B virus.

Epidemiology

Endemic in certain geographical areas where it may have been acquired perinatally. In western countries, it is spread sexually, particularly by homosexual anal intercourse, or parenterally as, for example, in i.v. drug misusers. Individuals whose serum contains e antigen are the most infectious.

Clinical features

Symptomless acute infections are common. Some persons develop acute icteric hepatitis after a prepatent period of 30–130 days. In a small proportion of patients, chronicity develops. Many of these individuals are well, without biochemical abnormalities of liver function. In others, chronic persistent or active hepatitis, cirrhosis or hepatocellular carcinoma may develop.

Sero-conversion from e antigenaemia to anti-e may occur eventually.

In chronic hepatitis B, although anti-HBc IgG is detected, anti-HBc IgM is not found.

Treatment

That of acute illness is symptomatic. There may be a role for interferon in chronic hepatitis.

Prevention

Vaccine should be offered to those at risk.

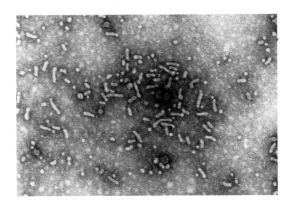

Fig. 79 Hepatitis B virus particles.

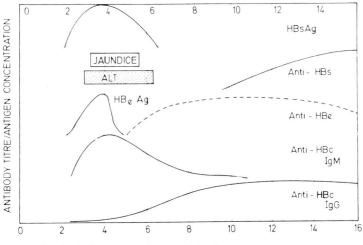

Fig. 80 Serological responses in acute infection.

12 | Epstein Barr Virus and Cytomegalovirus

Epstein Barr Virus (EBV)

Clinical features

This herpes virus is present in saliva and can be transmitted by kissing. Its presence in cervical epithelial cells suggests that it can be acquired also by sexual intercourse.

The virus is usually acquired in childhood when infection is inapparent. When infection is delayed until adolescence or early adulthood 50% of individuals develop the clinical features of infectious mononucleosis, malaise, fever, sore throat with a pharyngeal exudate, a maculopapular skin rash, generalised lymph-node enlargement, splenomegaly, sometimes mild icterus, and features of meningism. These features usually resolve within about 2 weeks, but a protracted illness may occur.

Diagnosis

The diagnosis is suggested by finding an absolute lymphocytosis with many atypical or pleomorphic cells; a finding of heterophil antibodies detected by the monospot slide test confirms the diagnosis.

Cytomegalovirus (CMV)

Cytomegalovirus can be transmitted hetero- and homosexually, vertically to the fetus, by breast and milk, or possibly by kissing.

Clinical features

Primary infection is usually symptomless, but a mononucleosis-like illness may develop: in this case however, the monospot test is negative. In immunodeficient individuals, e.g. people with AIDS, retinitis, pneumonia or colitis may occur. Congenital infection may produce no obvious effects, mental retardation, or be associated with the classical features of microcephaly, hepatosplenomegaly, chorioretinitis, uveitis or purpura.

Diagnosis

Diagnosis is by culture of the virus or from the urine or pharyngeal secretions or by serology.

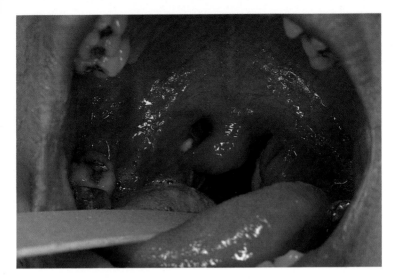

Fig. 81 Pharyngitis of EBV.

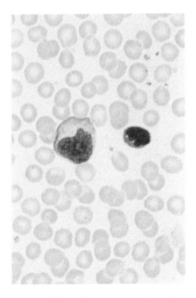

Fig. 82 Blood film from patient with acute mononucleosis.

13 | Human Immunodeficiency Virus Infection (1)

Aetiology

The human immunodeficiency viruses (HIV) are RNA-containing retroviruses that attack cells that bear the CD4 antigen-lymphocytes, macrophages, Langerhan's cells, microglia and other cells including natural killer cells, and interfere with cellular immunity. There is a progressive decrease in the number of CD4 cells in the peripheral blood. Polyclonal B cell activation with hypergammaglobulinaemia and impaired humoral immune responses are also features. Within 10 years 50% of individuals develop AIDS.

Epidemiology

The viruses that are present in blood, semen and cervicovaginal secretions, can be transmitted sexually—both homo- and heterosexually, by transfusion of contaminated blood or by contaminated syringes and needles. Concurrent sexually transmitted disease may facilitate sexually transmitted HIV infection. They can be transmitted also to the fetus from an infected mother. Infectivity increases as the duration of the infection increases.

Prevalence of HIV 1 infection varies geographically but is high in some areas (e.g. Central Africa) and in some groups (e.g. i.v. drug misusers in the Scottish capital Edinburgh). The incidence of infection may be decreasing in homosexual men.

HIV 2 is endemic in West Africa.

Clinical features

Most HIV-infected persons are symptomless. Shortly before seroconversion a small proportion develop a mononucleosis-like illness with abrupt onset of fever, headache, arthralgia, myalgia, diarrhoea, a maculopapular skin rash, generalised lymphadenopathy, aphthous ulceration of the mouth or candidiasis. Meningo-encephalitis may occur. These features usually resolve within about 2 weeks.

SEXUALLY TRANSMITTED DISEASES

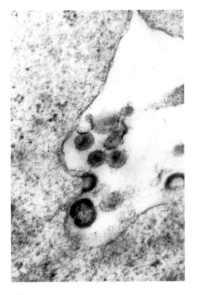

Fig. 83 Electron photomicrograph of HIV 1.

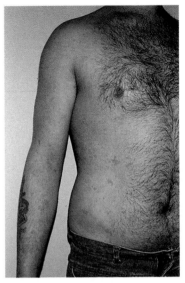

Fig. 84 Rash associated with seroconversion.

Fig. 85 Rash associated with seroconversion.

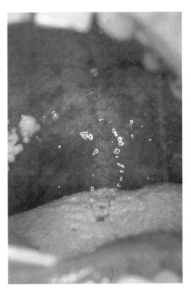

Fig. 86 Oral candidiasis with seroconversion.

Human Immunodeficiency Virus Infection (2)

Persistent generalised lymphadenopathy (PGL) is common and defined as enlargement (1 cm in diameter) of lymph nodes in at least two non-contiguous sites excluding inguinal, for at least 3 months; other causes of lymphadenopathy are excluded. The enlargement is usually symptomless. Nodes are firm, mobile, discrete and non-tender. Histologically there is usually reactive hyperplasia; involution may herald onset of secondary infections. In an HIV seropositive individual, biopsy is not indicated unless there is doubt about the diagnosis, and lymphoma or infections such as tuberculosis are considered.

Skin lesions are frequent in persons with PGL. Few of these are specific for HIV, but they are often more extensive and recalcitrant to treatment than in immunocompetent individuals. Lesions include seborrhoeic dermatitis of the face, chest and upper arms; folliculitis of the beard area, chest, arms and thighs; multiple molluscum contagiosum; extensive tinea pedis and cruris; frequently recurring HSV infection; multiple dermatomal herpes zoster; recalcitrant anogenital warts; xeroderma. Purpura may be a feature of thrombocytopenia.

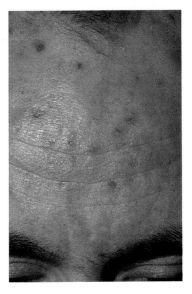

Fig. 87 Seborrhoeic dermatitis of forehead.

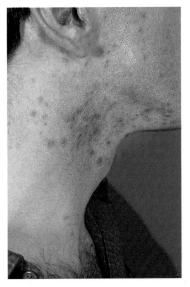

Fig. 88 Folliculitis of the beard area.

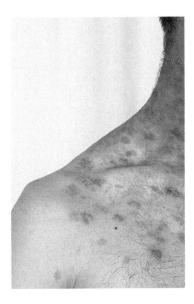

Fig. 89 Herpes zoster.

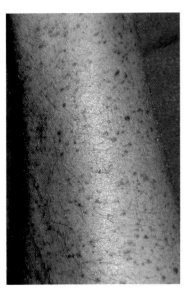

Fig. 90 Thrombocytopaenic purpura.

Human Immunodeficiency Virus Infection (3)

Clinical features (contd)

Oral hairy leukoplakia affects the lateral borders of the tongue; candidiasis, angular cheilitis and erosive gingivitis and aphthous ulceration are other oral manifestations.

Additional features that herald the onset of serious disease include weight loss, febrile episodes, night sweats, persistent diarrhoea and lethargy. Features of dementia may also develop.

Some of the infections and neoplasia that are indicative of cellular immunodeficiency and permit a diagnosis of AIDS are considered on pp. 63–70.

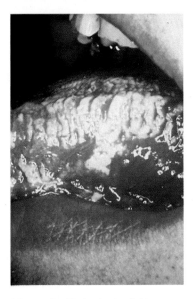

Fig. 91 Oral hairy leukoplakia.

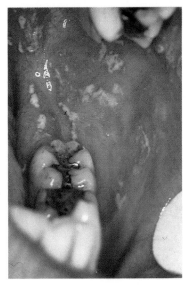

Fig. 92 Oral candidiasis.

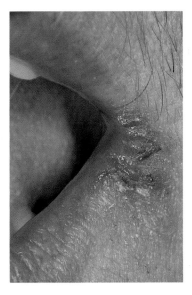

Fig. 93 Angular cheilitis.

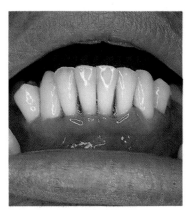

Fig. 94 Gingivitis.

Human Immunodeficiency Virus Infection (4)

Protozoal infections

Pneumocystis carinii is the most common opportunistic infection in AIDS. The pneumonia presents as increasing dyspnoea, non-productive cough and chest pain. In the early stages, there may be few signs; later, widespread coarse crepitations may be heard. Chest X-ray may be normal or show diffuse shadowing. Diagnosis is by the detection of cysts in induced sputum, bronchio-alveolar washings, or in biopsy material. Treatment is with intravenous cotrimoxazole or pentamidine. Skin rashes with leucopaenia or thrombocytopenia are common with the former drug. After resolution prophylactic treatment is advised.

Toxoplasma gondii infestation can be disseminated or present as a cerebral abscess, with focal features. Diagnosis is by serology and imaging procedures. Findings in the latter are non-specific but allow a tentative diagnosis to be made. Treatment is with sulphamethoxazole and pyrimethamine. Prophylactic treatment is recommended after resolution of infestation.

Cryptosporidium spp affects the intestinal mucosa and causes severe diarrhoea. Diagnosis is made by finding oocysts in faeces or biopsy material. Currently there is no specific therapy.

Isospora belli is another cause of diarrhoea.

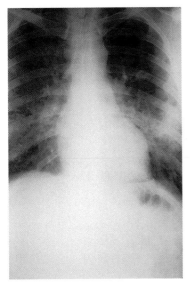

Fig. 95 *Pneumocystis carinii* pneumonia.

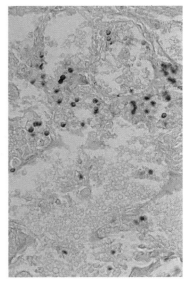

Fig. 96 *Pneumocystis carinii* in a lung biopsy.

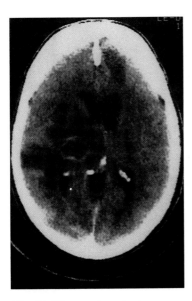

Fig. 97 CT scan of cerebral toxoplasmosis.

Fig. 98 Cryptosporidum oocysts in faeces.

13 | Human Immunodeficiency Virus Infection (5)

Bacterial infections

Mycobacterium tuberculosis may cause pulmonary disease alone or can be disseminated. Treatment is with standard anti-tuberculous therapy.

Atypical mycobacteria are associated with disseminated infection involving multiple organs. The intestinal tract may be severely affected. Diagnosis is made by detection of the organism in sputum, faeces, other body fluids or in biopsy material. There is no effective therapy at present.

Streptococcus pneumoniae and *Haemophilus influenzae* are causes of pneumonia. Diagnosis is by the detection of the bacteria in sputum or broncho-alveolar lavage. Treatment is with an antibiotic to which the isolate is sensitive.

Campylobacter spp can cause diarrhoea. Bacteria may be difficult to find in faeces and colonic biopsy may be necessary. Erythromycin or tetracyclines are used in treatment.

Shigella spp, especially *S. flexneri*, cause diarrhoea and bacteraemia is common. Recurrent infection is common. Diagnosis is by culture of faeces and blood. Treatment is with an appropriate antibiotic.

Salmonella enteritidis and *typhimurium* can cause diarrhoea and bacteraemia. Diagnosis is by culture of blood and faeces. Treat with an antibiotic to which the isolate is sensitive. As recurrence is very common, prophylaxis should be considered.

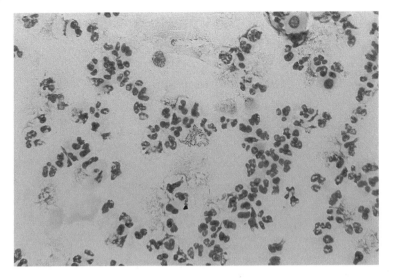

Fig. 99 Ziehl-Neelsen-stained smear of sputum showing *M. tuberculosis*.

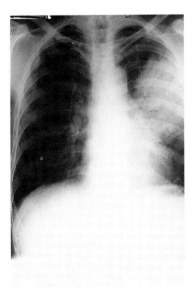

Fig. 100 Lobar pneumonia.

Human Immunodeficiency Virus Infection (6)

Fungal infections

Candida spp. Extensive superficial infection of mucosal surfaces is common. Oesophageal disease may cause dysphagia. Chronic vulvovaginitis is often troublesome. Dissemination is rare, but cerebral abscesses can occur. Treatment is with oral fluconazole and topical antifungal preparations. Prophylactic treatment is usually necessary.

Cryptococcus neoformans is the commonest cause of meningitis in patients with AIDS. There may be a few clinical features of the meningitis. Diagnosis is by finding yeasts in the CSF. Amphotericin B and 5-flucytosine or fluconazole are used in treatment.

Viral infections

Cytomegalovirus (CMV) is very common, but isolation from clinical material does not necessarily indicate a pathogenic role in a disease process. Often disseminated, CMV can cause colitis, pneumonia and retinitis.

Ganciclovir and foscarnet are useful in treatment, but relapse is common.

Herpes simplex virus can cause extensive ulceration of the anogenital tract and facial region. Acyclovir is very helpful in treatment and prophylaxis.

JC virus is associated with progressive multifocal leucoencephalopathy, a cause of dementia. Diagnosis is made by diagnostic imaging and biopsy.

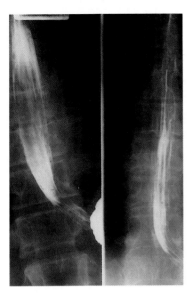

Fig. 101 Barium swallow showing oesophageal candidiasis.

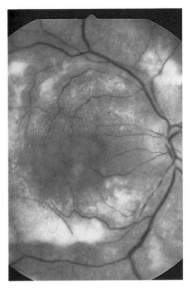

Fig. 102 CMV retinitis.

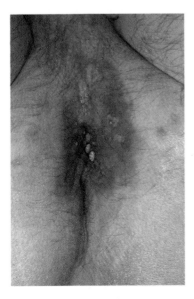

Fig. 103 Extensive perianal herpes.

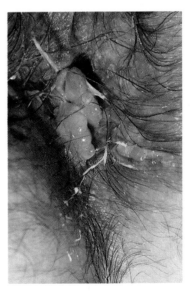

Fig. 104 Oedematous perianal skin tags in association with HSV.

Human Immunodeficiency Virus Infection (7)

Neoplasms

Kaposi's sarcoma is a tumour that probably arises from lymphatic endothelium. It is recognised in about 25% of homosexual men with AIDS, but is uncommon in other groups. The lesions are painless and non-pruritic, multiple, affecting any area of the body, including the head and neck. Mucosal involvement and visceral spread are common. Localised lesions may not require treatment unless they are on the face or in the oral cavity, when they may respond to chemotherapy. Radiotherapy to tumours of the feet that may produce severe oedema is indicated.

B-cell lymphomas, particularly extranodal and commonly affecting the gastrointestinal tract or brain, may develop. They are usually high-grade and when disseminated, respond poorly to chemotherapy.

Squamous-cell carcinomas of the anus and tongue have been reported.

AIDS in children

Usually developing within 2 years of birth, it presents with opportunistic infections, lymphoid interstitial pneumonitis and encephalopathy.

HIV encephalopathy

Subcortical dementia can be a late feature of HIV infection, even in the absence of other causes. There are signs of progressive cognitive and motor impairment. CT scanning or magnetic resonance imaging (MRI) show cortical atrophy, sometimes with parenchymal lesions.

Other neurological features include recurrent meningitis, vacuolar myelopathy, peripheral neuropathy, and myositis.

SEXUALLY TRANSMITTED DISEASES

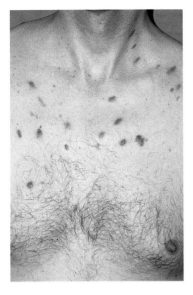

Fig. 105 Disseminated Kaposi's sarcoma.

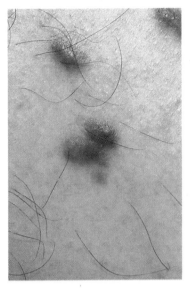

Fig. 106 Nodular lesion.

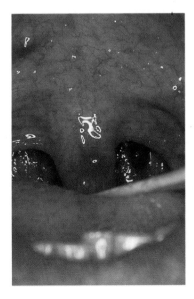

Fig. 107 Oral lesion.

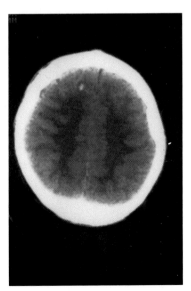

Fig. 108 CT scan showing cerebral atrophy.

Human Immunodeficiency Virus Infection (8)

Diagnosis

Serology. Elisa methods for antibodies against envelope proteins are used for screening, positive results being confirmed by another test, e.g. Western blot or competitive radioimmunoassay.

These antibodies become detectable at a very variable interval from infection, the average interval being about 3 months. The more sensitive polymerase chain reaction (PCR) to detect viral nucleic acids may prove to be a better diagnostic test.

HIV core antigen can be detected in the peripheral blood early in infection, but becomes undetectable as antibody develops. Later, antigen may again be found preceding the development of serious disease. At this time, core antibodies decline.

The diagnosis of HIV infection in children can be difficult. Maternal antibodies can persist for many months, there may be no detectable antibody response, and antigen is not always found; PCR may prove useful in diagnosis.

Treatment

Zidovudine is the only drug that is currently used in patients with AIDS or severe HIV-related features. In some patients improvement is not maintained. Side effects include a macrocytic anaemia and leucopaenia and a myositis.

Prevention

In the absence of an effective vaccine, control of infection depends on health education, e.g. encouraging the adoption of safer sexual practices and the avoidance of sharing non-sterile needles/syringes.

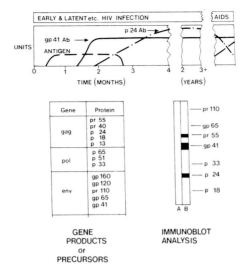

Gene	Protein
gag	pr 55 pr 40 p 24 p 18 p 13
pol	p 65 p 51 p 33
env	gp 160 gp 120 pr 110 gp 65 gp 41

GENE
PRODUCTS
or
PRECURSORS

IMMUNOBLOT
ANALYSIS

Fig. 109 Serological responses in HIV infection.

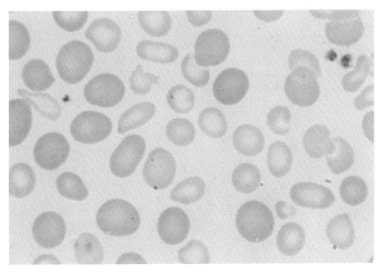

Fig. 110 Macrocytic anaemia associated with zidovudine therapy.

14 | Genital Candidiasis

Aetiology

Genital candidiasis is caused by species of yeasts, especially *Candida albicans*. These are found as saprophytes in the mouth, faeces and vagina. Conditions that favour transition from saprophyte to pathogen include pregnancy, tissue maceration, diabetes mellitus, antimicrobial agents, immunosuppressive drugs and HIV infection.

Clinical features

Intense pruritus vulvae is the most common symptom in the female. Other features include dyspareunia, vulval burning and swelling. There is marked redness of the inner aspects of the labia minora and vestibule sometimes extending to the labia majora, perineum and perianal skin. White plaques of variable size are found in the vagina which may be reddened. Primary cutaneous candidiasis affects the outer labia majora and genitocrural folds and presents as a weeping erythematous area with a scaly margin and small satellite pustules. In the male, there is soreness or itching of the penis with a subpreputial discharge. The glans and mucosal surface of the prepuce are inflamed with superfical erosions and preputial oedema. A similar picture may result from hypersensitivity to candidal antigens and develop within 6–24 hours of intercourse with an infected partner.

Diagnosis

Pseudohyphae in Gram-stained smears, or culture on a glucose peptone agar (Sabouraud's).

Treatment

Antifungal imidazoles (e.g. clotrimazole) as cream or pessaries. Partners may also need to be treated.

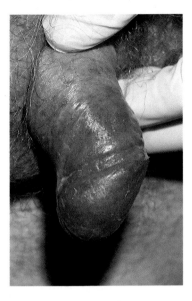

Fig. 111 Candidal balanoposthitis.

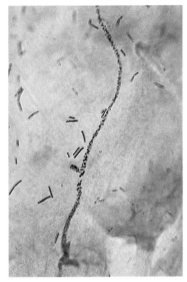

Fig. 112 Pseudohyphae of Candida species.

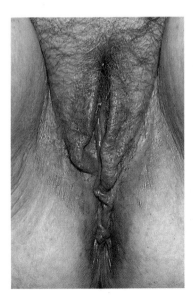

Fig. 113 Candidal vulvitis.

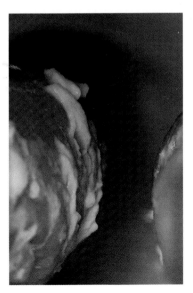

Fig. 114 Candidal vaginitis.

15 | Trichomoniasis

Aetiology

Trichomonas vaginalis is a flagellated protozoon that invades the superficial epithelial cells of the vagina, urethra, glans penis, prostate and seminal vesicles.

Epidemiology

The organism is almost always sexually transmitted but, rarely, female neonates can be infected during delivery. In the UK incidence has been decreasing. Concurrent sexually transmitted infections are common.

Clinical features

In the female, the most common symptoms are vaginal discharge with an unpleasant odour, vulval soreness, dyspareunia and dysuria. Some women are symptomless. There is a variable degree of vaginitis and vulvitis. The vaginal discharge is also variable, the classical frothy yellow discharge being found in less than one-third of infested women. Most infested men are symptomless, but urethritis and balanoposthitis may occur.

Diagnosis

Trichomonads may be found by direct microscopy or culture of vaginal exudate, or in the male, of urethral scrapings, prostatic fluid or centrifuged deposit of urine. The protozoon is sometimes found in Papanicolaou-stained cytology preparations. Specimens that cannot be examined immediately should be sent to the laboratory in a transport medium (e.g. Amies).

Treatment

Metronidazole is the treatment of choice. Although rare, resistance to this drug has been reported. Regular partners should be examined and treated. During treatment with metronidazole, alcohol should be avoided.

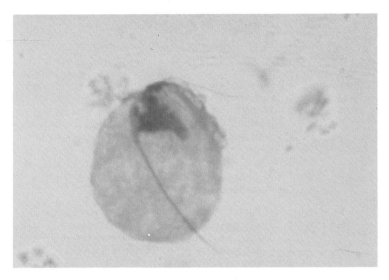

Fig. 115 *Trichomonas vaginalis* (Giemsa stain).

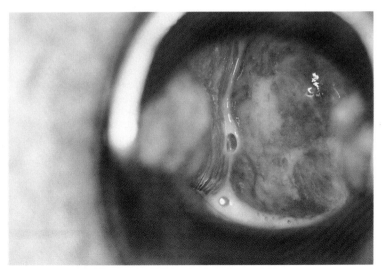

Fig. 116 Trichomonal vaginitis.

16 | Bacterial Vaginosis

Aetiology

Although no single bacterium is responsible, *Gardnerella vaginalis* and anaerobes such as *Mobiluncus spp*, peptostreptococci and *Bacteroides spp* (except *B. fragilis*) are associated with this clinical entity. The diamines putrescine and cadaverine and gamma-amino-n-butyric acid produced by the anaerobes are found in the vaginal discharge. Sexual transmission is possible.

Clinical features

The patient complains of an increased vaginal discharge with a fishy odour that is most noticeable during and after sexual intercourse. Pruritus vulvae is not a feature. There is a homogeneous grey-white discharge that may coat the vaginal walls and pool in the posterior fornix. Although the mucosa may be mildly oedematous, vaginitis is not a feature.

Diagnosis

Diagnosis is by recognition of the clinical features. The pH of infected vaginal secretions is higher than normal, generally >5.0. A characteristic odour is produced on mixing a drop of vaginal secretion and KOH on a slide. Infection produces a positive 'sniff test'. 'Clue cells' can be seen in a saline mount of secretion. In a Gram-stained smear, there are few bacteria of the *Lactobacillus* morphotype, but increased numbers of small Gram-negative rods. Other forms of Gram-negative rods and Gram-positive cocci are also found.

Treatment

Metronidazole is an effective short-term treatment. Relapse, however, is common. Treatment of partner may be indicated when there has been relapse.

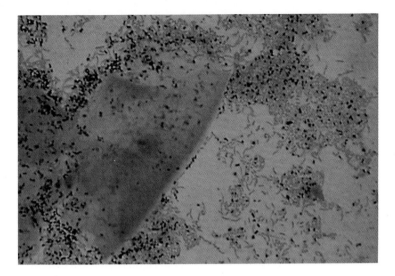

Fig. 117 Gram-stained smear of bacterial vaginosis.

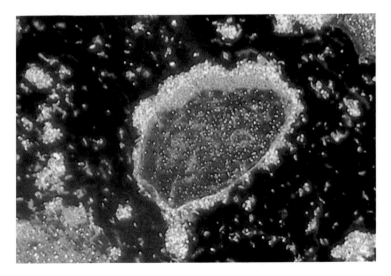

Fig. 118 Dark-field appearance of wet mount of vaginal material from bacterial vaginosis.

17 | Enteric Infections in Homosexual Men

Aetiology

Although playing a small part in the global epidemiology of these infections, the sexual transmission of enteric pathogens amongst homosexual men is important. Oro-anal contact is the principal means of acquisition of these organisms that include bacteria (*Shigella spp*, *Salmonella spp*, *Campylobacter spp*), viruses (hepatitis A, coronaviruses), protozoa (*Giardia intestinalis*, *Entamoeba histolytica*) and nematodes (*Enterobius vermicularis*). Symptomless carriers are important.

Clinical features

In immunocompetent men, the bacterial infections may be symptomless or cause an acute self-limiting diarrhoeal illness; in AIDS patients a more prolonged and severe illness may occur. A panproctocolitis is noted. Coronaviruses may be associated with diarrhoea and hepatitis A with acute icteric hepatitis. Although a proctocolitis with diarrhoea may result from *E. histolytica* infestation, most homosexual men are infested with a non-pathogenic stock of the amoeba. *Giardia* affects the upper small intestine, sometimes producing diarrhoea with features of malabsorption. Enterobiasis is often associated with pruritus ani.

Diagnosis

Diagnosis is achieved by the following approaches:
1. Bacterial infections by faecal cultures;
2. Hepatitis A by serology and coronaviruses by electron microscopy;
3. Protozoa by microscopy of faeces for cysts and trophozoites (jejunal fluid and biopsy are sometimes used for diagnosis of giardiasis;
4. *E. vermicularis* by Sellotape-strip microscopy.

Treatment

Specific chemotherapy when indicated.

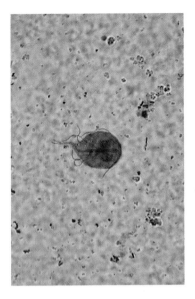

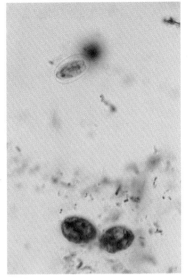

Fig. 119 Trophozoite of *Giardia intestinalis.*

Fig. 120 Cysts of *Giardia intestinalis*

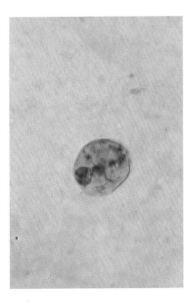

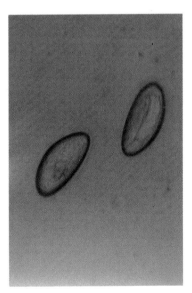

Fig. 121 Trophozoite of *Entamoeba histolytica.*

Fig. 122 Ova of *Enterobius vermicularis.*

18 | Pthiriasis

Aetiology

Pthirus pubis (crab louse) infests the strong hairs of the body-pubic and perianal areas, those of the thighs, legs, forearms, axillae, chest and, less frequently, eyelashes, eyebrows and beard. Eggs are laid at the bases of the hairs and after hatching the nymphs undergo three moults before maturity is reached, usually 3 weeks from oviposition.

Epidemiology

P. pubis is transmitted by close contact, particularly during sexual intercourse. As the louse may survive away from the body for up to 44 hours depending on conditions, transmission by fomites may rarely be possible. In the UK the prevalence has increased over the past decade.

Clinical features

Although many individuals are symptomless, pruritus in the pubic area is the most common feature. Rarely, bluish macules are seen on the trunk at the site of bites (maculae caeruleae). Pyoderma may result from scratching.

Treatment

Malathion (1%) or carbaryl (1%) lotions are useful in that both are lethal to lice and eggs. Petroleum jelly applied twice daily is used to treat eyelash infestation.

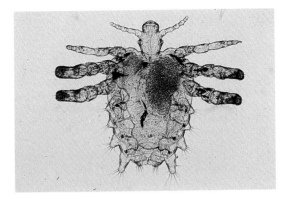

Fig. 123 *Pthirus pubis*: adult female.

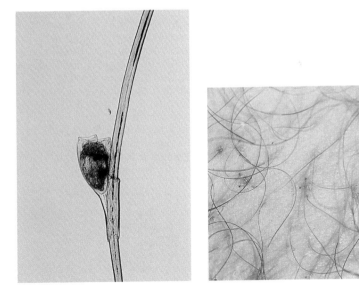

Fig. 124 *Pthirus pubis*: egg.

Fig. 125 Pthiriasis of pubic hair.

19 | Scabies

Aetiology

Caused by the mite *Sarcoptes scabiei* that burrows down into the stratum corneum where the female lays her eggs. These hatch and the larva leaves the burrow to find a new area of skin into which it burrows.

Epidemiology

Personal contact including sexual intercourse is the most usual means of acquisition of the parasite. Household spread is recognised also.

Clinical features

Four to six weeks after exposure, or earlier if there has been a previous infestation, the patient develops itch, particularly on retiring at night. The skin rash is roughly symmetrically distributed and is composed of burrows, that may be found on the finger webs and sides of the digits, flexor surfaces of the wrists and the penis, and papules that are seen on these areas and on the extensor surfaces of the elbows, anterior axillary folds, female breasts, abdomen, scrotum, lower buttocks and upper thighs. Papules may become excoriated and eczematous changes are common. Reddish-brown pruritic nodules that may persist for months even after treatment may be found on the elbows, axillary folds and male genitalia. In clean persons, lesions are often sparse. Secondary infection may occur.

Diagnosis

Mites and eggs found in skin scrapings.

Treatment

Lindane and benzyl benzoate are effective. The itch may persist for several weeks.

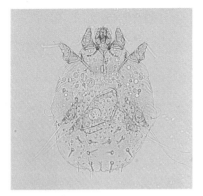

Fig. 126 Mite of *Sarcoptes scabiei*.

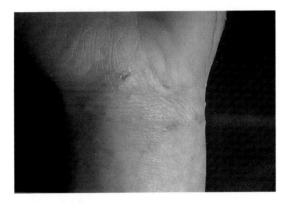

Fig. 127 Scabetic burrows.

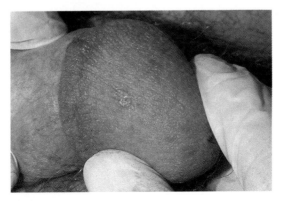

Fig. 128 Scabetic papules on the penis.

20 | Chancroid

Caused by *Haemophilus ducreyi*, this is an ulcerative condition of the genitalia, that is found mostly in tropical countries.

Clinical features

Single or multiple painful, tender superficial ulcers develop within a week of exposure. Phimosis may result from the inflammation. Inguinal lymph nodes on one or both sides enlarge and may suppurate, with the development of a unilocular abscess (bubo), that may rupture forming a sinus.

Diagnosis

The diagnosis is made by Gram-smear microscopy and culture of material from the edge of the ulcer. Treatment is with Augmentin, a cephalosporin or cotrimoxazole.

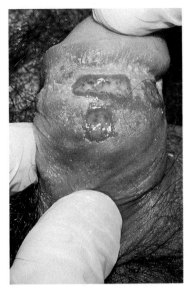

Fig. 129 Subpreputial chancroid.

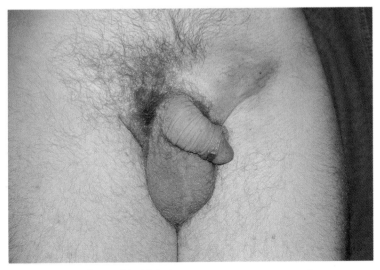

Fig. 130 Penile chancroid with bubo.

21 | Granuloma Inguinale (Donovanosis)

Aetiology

This is caused by the bacterium *Calymmato-bacterium granulomatis*. As it predominantly affects the genitalia, granuloma inguinale is thought to be sexually transmitted although this has not been proved conclusively. The condition is seen mainly in the tropics.

Clinical features

The prepatent period may be from 3 days to 6 months. The earliest lesion is a flat-topped papule which soon ulcerates. The ulcer spreads slowly along skin folds and the base may become elevated above the surrounding tissue. Extensive scarring occurs in some patients, especially women, in whom vulval oedema occurs. Extra genital sites are sometimes affected. Cancer may supervene later.

Diagnosis

On Giemsa staining of ulcer tissue, the bacteria are seen in mononuclear cells as the so-called Donovan bodies.

Treatment

This is usually with either tetracyclines or cotrimoxazole.

SEXUALLY TRANSMITTED DISEASES

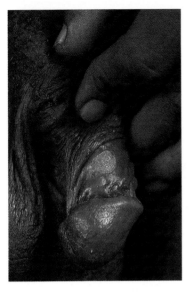 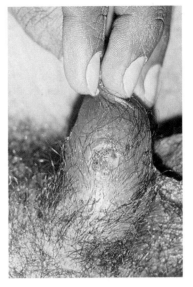

Fig. 131 Granuloma inguinale of penis.

Fig. 132 Granuloma inguinale of penis.

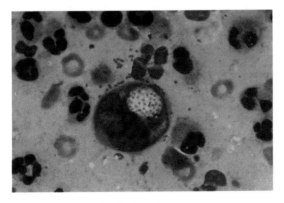

Fig. 133 Donovan bodies in a tissue smear.

22 | Lymphogranuloma Venereum (LGV)

Aetiology

Lymphogranuloma venereum (LGV) is caused by the L1−3 serovars of *Chlamydia trachomatis*. Most cases are found in the tropics.

Clinical features

A primary lesion is noticed by only one-third of those infected. After 3 days to 3 weeks, the lesion begins as a small painless papule which ulcerates and then heals after a few days. Thereafter, the patient develops tender, inguinal lymphadenopathy which is unilateral in two-thirds of cases. Abscesses (buboes) may form, and these may rupture resulting in sinus formation. The development of multiple buboes above and below Roupart's ligament may give 'the sign of the groove'.

Anorectal infection may result in an acute ulcerative proctitis.

Chronic vulval ulceration (esthiomene) and genital elephantiasis are uncommon later complications.

Diagnosis

Culture for *C. trachomatis* may be attempted from aspirated bubo pus. Serological tests may also be used.

Treatment

Tetracyclines such as doxycycline are usually given. Alternatives are erythromycin and rifampicin. Buboes should be aspirated to prevent rupture and sinus formation.

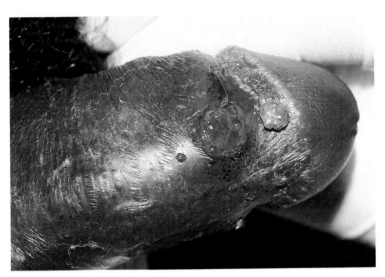

Fig. 134 Subpreputial ulcer of LGV.

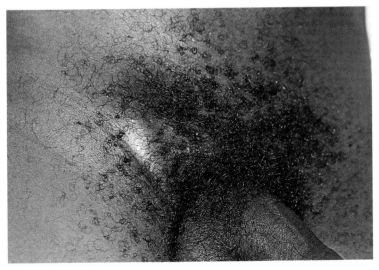

Fig. 135 Bubo of LGV.

23 | **Endemic Treponematoses**

Yaws

Caused by *Treponema pallidum ssp pertenue*, and found in the tropics, yaws is acquired during childhood by direct personal contact. After a prepatent period of 2 weeks to 3 months, a primary vegetative lesion develops that heals usually after several months leaving a hypopigmented scar. Secondary features that then develop include widespread raised, crusted papules particularly noticeable around orifices. Hyperkeratotic plaques develop on the feet. Lesions heal after several months and tertiary features develop 3–5 years later and include hyperkeratotic lesions on the palms and soles, subcutaneous ulcerative gummata occur and periostitis and osteitis of the long bones and facial structures can result in gross deformity. Treatment is with penicillin, and preventitive programmes are well-established in many areas.

Pinta

Caused by *T. pallidum ssp carateum*, and found in Central and South America, this disease is acquired by direct skin contact. Only the skin is affected, with the appearance of dyschromic and hyperkeratotic lesions.

Endemic syphilis

Occurring in the Middle East and Africa, this presents early as a mucocutaneous eruption, and later with destructive skin and bone lesions.

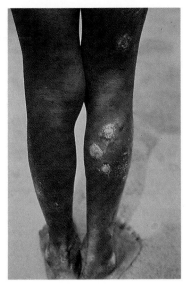

Fig. 136 Yaws: early.

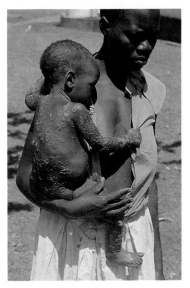

Fig. 137 Yaws: early.

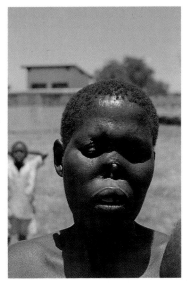

Fig. 138 Yaws: late Goundou.

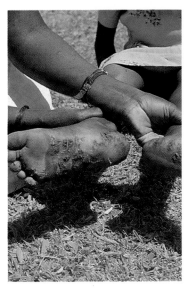

Fig. 139 Yaws: late lesions.

24

Infective Conditions of the Genitalia

Balanoposthitis

Common in uncircumcised men and often associated with anaerobic infections, but it can be a feature of contact dermatitis or allergic contact dermatitis. There is pain or itch, and often a malodorous subpreputial discharge. The inner surface of the prepuce and glans are reddened and there is a purulent discharge in the preputial sac. There may be superficial ulceration and preputial oedema with phimosis. Inguinal lymphadenitis is common.

Saline lavage is helpful and in more severe cases cotrimoxazole or metronidazole is needed. The urine must always be tested for glycosuria.

Tinea cruris

Caused by a species of dermatophyte, the lesions are bilateral and extend down the thighs and on to the scrotum. The skin is reddened and scaly and the margins are sharp. Small satellite lesions are usual. Diagnosis is made by finding hyphae in KOH preparations of skin scrapings. Treatment is with a topical imidazole.

Erythrasma

Caused by *Corynebacterium minutissimum*, erythrasma presents as non-pruritic, irregularly-shaped but sharply marginated red to brown patches that later become scaly.

Uni- or bilateral lesions affect the thighs and scrotum. Topical imidazoles are effective.

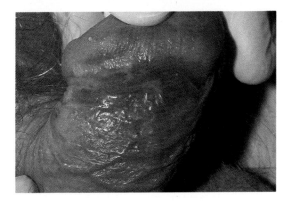

Fig. 140 Anaerobic balanoposthitis.

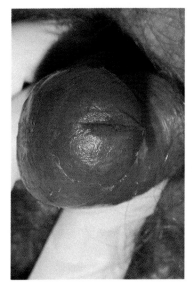

Fig. 141 Streptococcal balanoposthitis.

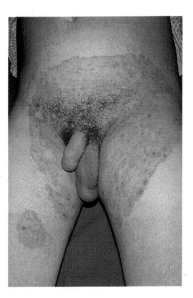

Fig. 142 Tinea cruris.

25

Genital Dermatoses

Psoriasis

Papules with scaling may be seen on the glans of the circumcised male. In the uncircumcised, the lesions are red with well-defined edges but there is no scaling. Other features are usually found, e.g. pitting of the nails. Diffuse plaques in the genitocrural folds or perianal region are red and sharply defined.

Lichen planus

Violaceous papules with flat shiny surfaces, less than 1 mm to more than 1 cm may be found on the external genitalia. Often symptomless, they may be pruritic. Linear lesions occur at the site of scratching and annular lesions are common on the penis. Lesions are self-limiting. In the buccal mucosa there may be a network of white streaks.

Eczema

The external genitalia may be involved in widespread eczema. Seborrhoeic dermatitis is usually flexural, the area being reddened with well-defined edges. Areas of lichenification (*lichen simplex*) may result from prolonged rubbing.

Irritant dermatitis

Painful reddened lesions with swelling and ulceration may follow contact with chemicals.

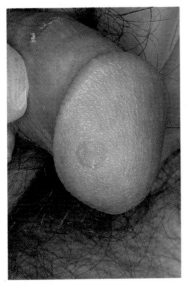

Fig. 143 Psoriasis of glans penis.

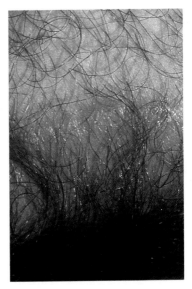

Fig. 144 Psoriasis of perianal region.

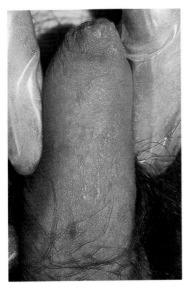

Fig. 145 Lichen planus of penis.

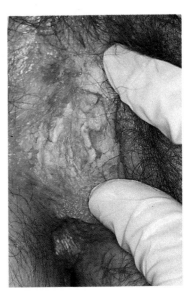

Fig. 146 Lichen simplex of vulva.

Genital Lesions in Systemic Disease (1)

Bullous erythema multiforme

Aetiology

Also known as Stevens-Johnson syndrome. This can be associated with viral (especially herpes simplex) and bacterial (especially *Mycoplasma pneumonae*) infections, drugs (such as sulphonamides) and collagen diseases; in more than 50% of cases there is no detectable precipitating factor.

Clinical features

Bullae develop suddenly on the oral and genital mucosae, ulcerate and become covered with a greyish white membrane; haemorrhagic crusting is common. There may be a marked conjunctivitis. Skin lesions that are not always present are dull-red maculopapules that may develop into target lesions, cropping at intervals of a few days is usual. The rash is found on the hands, wrists, forearms, elbows and knees.

Treatment

Treatment is symptomatic, but corticosteroids may be needed in severe cases. Recurrences can occur, particularly with herpetic infections.

Fixed drug eruption

Clinical features

These lesions recur in the same site each time the particular drug is given. The glans penis is a common site. There is an erythematous plaque that later darkens and is often surmounted by a bulla. Healing is accompanied by crusting and scaling. Residual pigmentation is common. Drugs that may be responsible include tetracycline, sulphonamides and barbiturates.

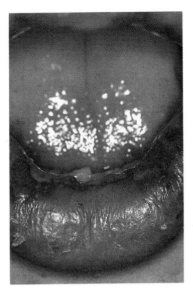

Fig. 147 Oral lesions of bullous erythema multiforme.

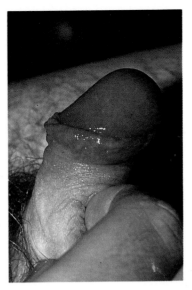

Fig. 148 Penile lesions of bullous erythema multiforme.

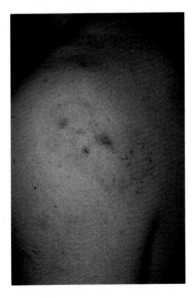

Fig. 149 Skin lesions of bullous erythema multiforme.

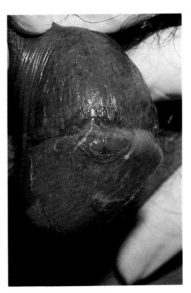

Fig. 150 Fixed drug eruption of the penis.

Genital Lesions in Systemic Disease (2)

Pyoderma gangrenosum

This condition can be associated with ulcerative colitis, rheumatoid arthritis and chronic suppurative conditions. The characteristic lesion is an irregular ulcer with a ragged, bluish and overhanging edge, and a necrotic base. Multiple ulcers are sometimes found. Treatment is symptomatic, but the ulceration can persist for years. Any underlying condition should be treated.

Crohn's disease

This may affect the anogenital region and present as vulval oedema, oedematous perianal skin tags, fistulae, abscesses and ulceration. Diagnosis is by histology. Differential diagnosis includes tuberculosis, lymphogranuloma venereum, malignancy, hidradenitis and deep fungal infection.

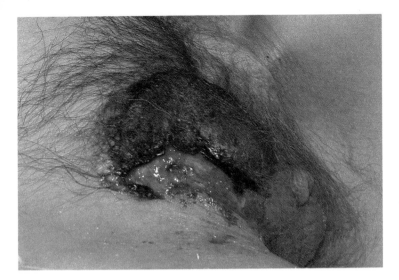

Fig. 151 Pyoderma gangrenosum of vulva.

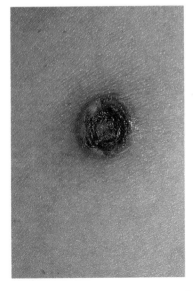

Fig. 152 Pyoderma gangrenosum of thigh.

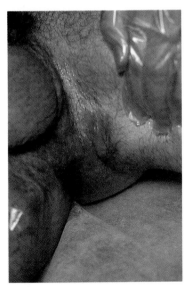

Fig. 153 Perianal Crohn's disease.

This is a multisystem disease characterised by oral, genital and ocular lesions with a tendency to exacerbations and remissions. It is of unknown aetiology but principally affects individuals of East Mediterranean or Japanese origin. The common histological feature is a vasculitis.

Clinical features

In the mucocutaneous form of the syndrome, there are recurrent multiple, painful ulcers of the oral mucosa. The lesions usually heal within 2 weeks but some may be persistent and heal with scarring. Similar ulceration of the genitalia may occur. Skin lesions include ulceration, pustules, erythema nodosum and erythema multiforme. The mucocutaneous signs may be the only features of Behçet's syndrome or may accompany or antedate other manifestations. Anterior uveitis, phlebitis, venous occlusion, macular or optic-disc oedema and vitreous cellular infiltration are the ocular features; blindness may result. In about 50% of cases, arthritis or arthralgia of the knees, ankles, wrists and elbows occurs. Neurological features include cranial nerve palsies, cerebellar and spinal cord lesions and meningoencephalitis.

Treatment

Oral and genital ulceration may respond to treatment with topical corticosteroids but ocular and visceral disease may require immunosuppressive chemotherapy.

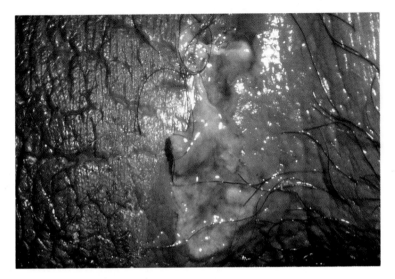

Fig. 154 Scrotal ulcer in Behçet's syndrome.

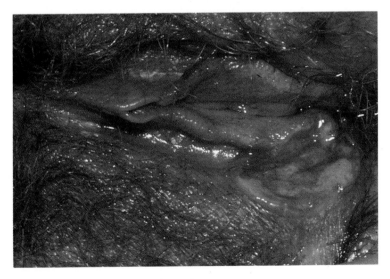

Fig. 155 Vulval ulcer in Behçet's syndrome.

28

Lichen Sclerosus et Atrophicus

Lichen sclerosus et atrophicus (LSA) is rare and affects women more frequently than men. The median age at onset is about 50 years in women and slightly earlier in men.

Clinical features

Vulval soreness and dyspareunia are the symptoms in females. The perianal region, inner aspects of the labia minora and vestibule are usually affected. Pearly-white atrophic papules with follicular plugging may be seen in the perianal region but on the vulva friction and moisture produce erosion of their surfaces resulting in a red, raw area. There is genital atrophy and the introitus is constricted. Haemorrhagic vesicles and telangiectatic lesions are common. Lichenification and small, deep fissures may result. Lesions may be found elsewhere on the body.

The glans penis and prepuce are the sites affected in the male. Phimosis is a feature and meatal stricture may ensue. The glans and mucosal surface of the prepuce are white, the surface often showing telangiectasia.

When the onset has been in middle age, the lesions are unlikely to remit. Leukoplakia and squamous cell carcinoma may complicate the condition.

Treatment

The treatment is symptomatic with bland creams or corticosteroid preparations. In the male there should be attention to hygiene. Circumcision and urethral meatotomy may be necessary.

Plasma cell balanitis

Of uncertain cause, this presents in older men as a chronic balanitis with a moist shiny surface stippled with 'cayenne pepper' spots. There is a poor response to any treatment.

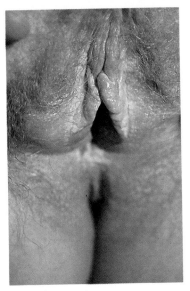

Fig. 156 LSA of vulva.

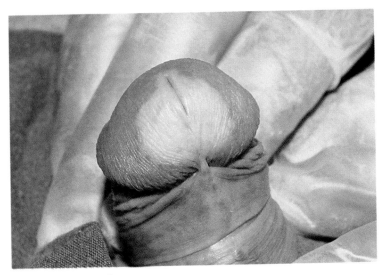

Fig. 157 LSA of penis.

29

Premalignant and Malignant Conditions

Intraepidermal carcinoma (Bowen's disease)

Middle-aged women are most commonly affected. The condition may progress to squamous cell carcinoma and be associated with malignancy elsewhere in the genital tract.

Pruritus vulvae or ani, or soreness are the symptoms. There is a well-demarcated red, slightly scaly and somewhat elevated plaque that slowly increases in size. Any part of the vulva can be involved. The diagnosis is made by histology. Surgical excision or topical application of 5-fluorouracil are used to treat the condition.

Erythroplasia of Queyrat

This premalignant condition occurs in men aged between 50 and 60 years. There is a very slightly elevated, soft, well-demarcated, bright-red velvety plaque that occurs on the glans penis or mucosal surface of the prepuce. It is slowly progressive. The diagnosis is made by biopsy. Treatment is by cryotherapy or the topical application of 5-fluorouracil.

Squamous cell carcinoma

On the penis the most common presentation is that of a warty lesion in the preputial sac; ulceration may occur later. Rarely, the locally invasive form (Buschke-Lowenstein) may occur. Vulval and anal lesions tend to be ulcerated. Other malignancies such as basal-cell carcinoma and melanoma are rare.

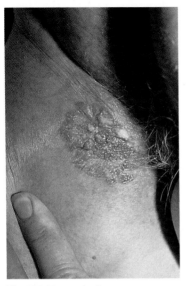

Fig. 158 Bowen's disease.

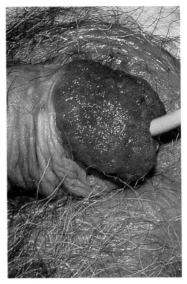

Fig. 159 Erythroplasia of Queyrat.

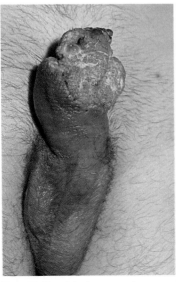

Fig. 160 Buschke-Lowenstein tumour.

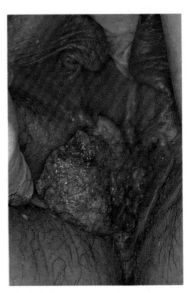

Fig. 161 Squamous cell carcinoma of the vulva.